Cardiac PET Imaging

Guest Editors

WENGEN CHEN, MD, PhD
AMOL M. TAKALKAR, MD, MS

PET CLINICS

www.pet.theclinics.com

Consulting Editor
ABASS ALAVI, MD, PhD (Hon), DSc (Hon)

October 2011 • Volume 6 • Number 4

SAUNDERS an imprint of ELSEVIER, Inc.

W.B. SAUNDERS COMPANY
A Division of Elsevier Inc.

1600 John F. Kennedy Boulevard • Suite 1800 • Philadelphia, Pennsylvania 19103-2899

http://www.theclinics.com

PET CLINICS Volume 6, Number 4
October 2011 ISSN 1556-8598, ISBN-13: 978-1-4557-1120-8

Editor: Barton Dudlick
Developmental Editor: Eva Kulig

PET Clinics (ISSN 1556-8598) is published quarterly by Elsevier Inc., 360 Park Avenue South, New York, NY 10010-1710. Months of issue are January, April, July, and October. Periodicals postage paid at New York, NY, and additional mailing offices. Subscription prices per year are $215.00 (US individuals), $297.00 (US institutions), $110.00 (US students), $244.00 (Canadian individuals), $332.00 (Canadian institutions), $124.00 (Canadian students), $260.00 (foreign individuals), $332.00 (foreign institutions), and $134.00 (foreign students). To receive student and resident rate, orders must be accompanied by name of affiliated institution, date of term, and the signature of program/residency coordinator on institution letterhead. Orders will be billed at individual rate until proof of status is received. Foreign air speed delivery is included in all Clinics subscription prices. All prices are subject to change without notice. POSTMASTER: Send address changes to PET Clinics, Elsevier Health Sciences Division, Subscription Customer Service, 3251 Riverport Lane, Maryland Heights, MO 63043. **Customer Service: 1-800-654-2452 (U.S. and Canada); 314-447-8871 (outside U.S. and Canada). Fax: 314-447-8029. E-mail: journalscustomerservice-usa@elsevier.com (for print support); journalsonlinesupport-usa@elsevier.com (for online support).**

Reprints. For copies of 100 or more of articles in this publication, please contact the Commercial Reprints Department, Elsevier Inc., 360 Park Avenue South, New York, NY 10010-1710. Tel.: 212-633-3812; Fax: 212-462-1935; E-mail: reprints@elsevier.com.

Printed and bound by CPI Group (UK) Ltd, Croydon, CR0 4YY

Transferred to Digital Print 2011

Contributors

CONSULTING EDITOR

ABASS ALAVI, MD, PhD (Hon), DSc (Hon)
Professor of Radiology, Division of Nuclear
Medicine, University of Pennsylvania School of
Medicine, Philadelphia, Pennsylvania

GUEST EDITORS

WENGEN CHEN, MD, PhD
Assistant Professor, Department of Diagnostic
Radiology and Nuclear Medicine, University of
Maryland School of Medicine, Baltimore,
Maryland

AMOL M. TAKALKAR, MD, MS
Medical Director, PET Imaging Center,
Biomedical Research Foundation of Northwest
Louisiana; Associate Professor of Clinical
Radiology, Associate Director of Research,
Department of Radiology, Louisiana State
University Health Sciences Center – Shreveport,
Shreveport, Louisiana

AUTHORS

ABDULRAHMAN ABDULBAKI, MD
Cardiology Division, Department of Internal
Medicine, Louisiana State University Health
Sciences Center – Shreveport, Shreveport,
Louisiana

ABASS ALAVI, MD, PhD (Hon), DSc (Hon)
Professor of Radiology, Division of Nuclear
Medicine, University of Pennsylvania School of
Medicine, Philadelphia, Pennsylvania

WENGEN CHEN, MD, PhD
Assistant Professor, Department of Diagnostic
Radiology and Nuclear Medicine, University of
Maryland School of Medicine, Baltimore,
Maryland

ALIN CHIRINDEL, MD
Department of Diagnostic Radiology and
Nuclear Medicine, University of Maryland
School of Medicine, Baltimore, Maryland

BENOIT DESJARDINS, MD, PhD
Assistant Professor, Department of Radiology,
University of Pennsylvania, Philadelphia,
Pennsylvania

TIMM DICKFELD, MD, PhD
Division of Cardiology, University of Maryland
School of Medicine, Baltimore, Maryland

VICTOR FERRARI, MD
Cardiovascular Division, Department of
Medicine, University of Pennsylvania,
Philadelphia, Pennsylvania

ARI GOLDBERG, MD, PhD
Geisinger Healthcare, Danville, Pennsylvania

GAGANDEEP S. GURM, MD
Cardiology Division, Department of Medicine,
Massachusetts General Hospital and Harvard
Medical School, Boston, Massachusetts

YUCHI HAN, MD, MMSc
Cardiovascular Division, Department of
Medicine, University of Pennsylvania,
Philadelphia, Pennsylvania

SAURABH JHA, MBBS
Assistant Professor of Radiology, Department
of Radiology, University of Pennsylvania
Medical Center, Philadelphia, Pennsylvania

ABIGAIL MAY KHAN, MD
Cardiovascular Division, Department of
Medicine, University of Pennsylvania,
Philadelphia, Pennsylvania

HAROLD LITT, MD, PhD
Department of Radiology, University of
Pennsylvania, Philadelphia, Pennsylvania

MINH LU, MD
Department of Diagnostic Radiology and
Nuclear Medicine, University of Maryland
School of Medicine, Baltimore, Maryland

KALGI MODI, MD, FACC
Cardiology Division, Department of Internal
Medicine, Louisiana State University Health
Sciences Center – Shreveport, Shreveport,
Louisiana

OLGA MOLCHANOVA-COOK, MD, PhD
Department of Diagnostic Radiology and
Nuclear Medicine, University of Maryland
School of Medicine, Baltimore, Maryland

BABAK SABOURY, MD, MPH
Post-Doctoral Clinical Research Fellow,
Department of Radiology, School of Medicine,
University of Pennsylvania, Philadelphia,
Pennsylvania

MARK F. SMITH, PhD
Department of Diagnostic Radiology and
Nuclear Medicine, University of Maryland
School of Medicine, Baltimore, Maryland

MARK STELLINGWORTH, MD
University Medical Center, Lafayette,
Louisiana

AMOL M. TAKALKAR, MD, MS
Medical Director, PET Imaging Center,
Biomedical Research Foundation of
Northwest Louisiana; Associate Professor of
Clinical Radiology, Associate Director of
Research, Department of Radiology,
Louisiana State University Health Sciences
Center – Shreveport, Shreveport, Louisiana

JING TIAN, MD, PhD
Division of Cardiology, University of Maryland
School of Medicine, Baltimore, Maryland

CHARLES S. WHITE, MD
Professor of Radiology and Medicine and
Chief of Thoracic Radiology, Department of
Diagnostic Radiology and Nuclear Medicine,
University of Maryland School of Medicine,
Baltimore, Maryland

POUYA ZIAI, MD
Research Scholar, Department of Radiology,
School of Medicine, University of
Pennsylvania, Philadelphia, Pennsylvania

Contents

and subsequent rupture. Several invasive and non-invasive structural imaging techniques have been utilized to diagnose atherosclerosis, but none of these methods are capable of detecting and quantifying molecular calcification. Fluorine-18-Sodium Fluoride (18F-NaF) positron emission tomography/computed tomography (PET/CT) imaging allows detection and quantification of arterial molecular calcification in heart and across multiple vessels. In this review the authors discuss the feasibility, application and potential future of 18F-NaF-PET/CT in detecting molecular calcification and in defining the future risk of atherosclerotic plaque rupture in the affected vessels.

Can Vascular Wall ^{18}F-FDG Uptake on PET Imaging Serve as a Biomarker of Vulnerable Atherosclerotic Plaque?

Wengen Chen

Vulnerable atherosclerotic plaques, which are highly inflammatory but not flow limiting, account for most cardiovascular events. Current cardiovascular imaging modalities are based on anatomic detection of artery luminal narrowing and are unable to detect vulnerable plaques. Preliminary data indicate the role of vascular FDG uptake as a biomarker of vulnerable plaque. Direct visualization of coronary artery plaques may become clinically feasible in the near future with the development of a PET/CT technology optimized for cardiovascular imaging, along with progress in standardization of cardiac PET imaging protocol, such as dietary preparation, acquisition mode, acquisition time after the injection of the radiotracer, and cardiac gating.

Role of Global Disease Assessment by Combined PET-CT-MR Imaging in Examining Cardiovascular Disease

Babak Saboury, Pouya Ziai, and Abass Alavi

Atherosclerosis is considered a chronic inflammatory disease, and thereafter the degree of this pathologic process is considered to be a major determinant in plaque stability and in forecasting future events. Over the past decade, ^{18}F-fluorodeoxyglucose PET/computed tomography has become a well-established imaging modality in evaluating various inflammatory disorders, and has been shown to be very useful in evaluating plaque activity in major arteries. This emerging noninvasive imaging modality has great potential in evaluating plaque vulnerability and in predicting the risk of future rupture and consequent thrombosis.

Relative Merits of Single-Photon Emission Computed Tomography and PET Perfusion Imaging: A Cardiologist's View

Abdulrahman Abdulbaki, Kalgi Modi, and Amol M. Takalkar

Evidence from the medical literature supports the use of Cardiac positron emission tomography (PET) scanning to assess myocardial viability in patients with severe Left ventricular dysfunction who are being considered for revascularization. Cardiac PET has emerged as an alternative to Single Photon Emission Computed Tomography (SPECT) imaging for assessment of Coronary Artery Disease. PET scanning is less likely than SPECT scanning to provide indeterminate results. The aim of the present paper is to review existing literature on relative merits of Cardiac PET imaging.

Recent advances in multidetector computed tomography (CT), with submillimeter spatial resolution, improved temporal resolution, and electrocardiographic gating, make it possible to image and accurately characterize the coronary arteries. Cardiac CT offers the ability to noninvasively assess cardiovascular anatomy, including coronary arteries, bypass grafts and stents, myocardium, pericardium, and cardiac function. A growing body of literature supports the prognostic value of coronary CT angiography. This article provides an overview of clinical applications, scanning protocols, limitations, and future developments of cardiac CT.

Coronary artery disease (CAD) is the leading cause of death in the adult population in the United States. Imaging is an essential component of the management of CAD, providing both diagnostic and prognostic information. This review provides an overview of the use of cardiovascular magnetic resonance (CMR) imaging in the evaluation of ischemia in both acute and chronic settings. The authors compare CMR imaging with other imaging modalities, highlighting the advantages and opportunities of CMR imaging, as well as limitations.

Cardiac magnetic resonance (CMR) imaging plays an important role in the distinction between ischemic and nonischemic cardiomyopathy. It does so principally by its excellent soft-tissue contrast and its ability to detect scar tissue. The distribution of scar tissue not only allows the diagnosis of coronary artery disease in a failing heart but also the type of nonischemic cardiomyopathy. The incorporation of CMR imaging early in the diagnostic cascade of a patient with heart failure of unknown cause can potentially avoid a cardiac catheterization.

This article reviews the increasing role of cardiac MR imaging to quantitatively assess myocardial scar in the context of clinical cardiac electrophysiology. After a quick overview of the biologic aspects of myocardial scar, two imaging techniques currently used to routinely image scar in cardiac electrophysiology contexts are described, MR imaging and electroanatomic mapping, and their relationship is explained. The main clinical issues involving MR imaging for cardiac electrophysiology are then reviewed, including imaging in cardiomyopathy (both ischemic and nonischemic), imaging for cardiac ablation therapy, and imaging of subjects with intracardiac devices.

PET Clinics

THE CLINICS ARE NOW AVAILABLE ONLINE!

Access your subscription at:
www.theclinics.com

GOAL STATEMENT

The goal of the *PET Clinics* is to keep practicing radiologists and radiology residents up to date with current clinical practice in positron emission tomography by providing timely articles reviewing the state of the art in patient care.

ACCREDITATION

PET Clinics is planned and implemented in accordance with the Essential Areas and Policies of the Accreditation Council for Continuing Medical Education (ACCME) through the joint sponsorship of the University of Virginia School of Medicine and Elsevier. The University of Virginia School of Medicine is accredited by the ACCME to provide continuing medical education for physicians.

The University of Virginia School of Medicine designates this enduring material activity for a maximum of 15 *AMA PRA Category 1 Credit(s)*™ *for each issue,* 60 credits per year. Physicians should only claim credit commensurate with the extent of their participation in the activity.

The American Medical Association has determined that physicians not licensed in the US who participate in this CME enduring material activity are eligible for a maximum of 15 *AMA PRA Category 1 Credit(s)*™ for each issue, 60 credits per year.

Credit can be earned by reading the text material, taking the CME examination online at http://www.theclinics.com/home/cme, and completing the evaluation. After taking the test, you will be required to review any and all incorrect answers. Following completion of the test and evaluation, your credit will be awarded and you may print your certificate.

FACULTY DISCLOSURE/CONFLICT OF INTEREST

The University of Virginia School of Medicine, as an ACCME accredited provider, endorses and strives to comply with the Accreditation Council for Continuing Medical Education (ACCME) Standards of Commercial Support, Commonwealth of Virginia statutes, University of Virginia policies and procedures, and associated federal and private regulations and guidelines on the need for disclosure and monitoring of proprietary and financial interests that may affect the scientific integrity and balance of content delivered in continuing medical education activities under our auspices.

The University of Virginia School of Medicine requires that all CME activities accredited through this institution be developed independently and be scientifically rigorous, balanced and objective in the presentation/discussion of its content, theories and practices.

All authors/editors participating in an accredited CME activity are expected to disclose to the readers relevant financial relationships with commercial entities occurring within the past 12 months (such as grants or research support, employee, consultant, stock holder, member of speakers bureau, etc.). The University of Virginia School of Medicine will employ appropriate mechanisms to resolve potential conflicts of interest to maintain the standards of fair and balanced education to the reader. Questions about specific strategies can be directed to the Office of Continuing Medical Education, University of Virginia School of Medicine, Charlottesville, Virginia.

The faculty and staff of the University of Virginia Office of Continuing Medical Education have no financial affiliations to disclose.

The authors/editors listed below have identified no professional or financial affiliations for themselves or their spouse/partner:

Abdulrahman Abdulbaki, MD; Abass Alavi, MD, PhD (Hon), DSc (Hon) (Consulting Editor); Sarah Barth, (Acquisitions Editor); Wengen Chen, MD, PhD (Guest Editor); Alin Chirindel, MD; Ari Goldberg, MD, PhD; Gagandeep S. Gurm, MD; Yuchi Han, MD, MMSc; Abigail May Khan, MD; Harold Litt, MD, PhD; Minh Lu, MD; Kalgi Modi, MD, FACC; Olga Molchanova-Cook, MD, PhD; Patrice Rehm, MD (Test Editor); Babak Saboury, MD, MPH; Mark Stellingworth, MD; Amol M. Takalkar, MD, MS (Guest Editor); Jing Tian, MD, PhD; and Charles S. White, MD; Pouya Ziai, MD.

The authors/editors listed below identified the following professional or financial affiliations for themselves or their spouse/partner:

Timm Dickfeld, MD, PhD is a consultant, and is on the Speakers' Bureau and is on the Advisory Board for Biosense.
Victor Ferrari, MD is on the Advisory Board for the Society for Cardiovascular Magnetic Resonance and the Journal of Cardiovascular Magnetic Resonance.
Saurabh Jha, MBBS receives research funding from General Electric.
Mark F. Smith, PhD is an industry funded researcher for GE Healthcare and Siemens Medical Solutions.

Disclosure of Discussion of Non-FDA Approved Uses for Pharmaceutical Products and/or Medical Devices

The University of Virginia School of Medicine, as an ACCME provider, requires that all faculty presenters identify and disclose any off-label uses for pharmaceutical and medical device products. The University of Virginia School of Medicine recommends that each physician fully review all the available data on new products or procedures prior to clinical use.

TO ENROLL

To enroll in the PET Clinics Continuing Medical Education program, call customer service at 1-800-654-2452 or visit us online at www.theclinics.com/home/cme. The CME program is available to subscribers for an additional fee of $196.00.

Preface
Cardiac PET Imaging

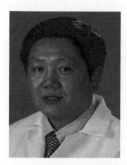 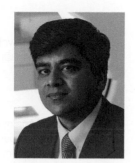

Wengen Chen, MD, PhD   Amol M. Takalkar, MD, MS
Guest Editors

Cardiovascular disease (CVD), more commonly referred to as "heart disease," is the number one killer in developed countries. Coronary heart disease causes approximately one of every six deaths in the United States.[1] In addition, CVD is also a primary cause of hospitalization and disability, resulting in a staggering cost burden to our society in the form of health expenditures and lost productivity.

Cardiovascular imaging modalities, such as coronary angiography and nuclear myocardial perfusion scan, play an important role in CVD diagnosis and management. These studies emphasize anatomical changes of coronary arteries, for example, luminal narrowing, and its downstream flow-limiting consequence in the left ventricular myocardium. Clinically, when CVD is diagnosed with these modalities, the underlying cause of the disease (usually atherosclerosis) has already progressed to its advanced stage. It is a laudable goal to develop a noninvasive imaging modality that can detect accurately and reliably the so-called "unstable plaque" believed to be the culprit lesion for most of the fatal cardiac events.[2] Studies have demonstrated the feasibility of characterization of coronary and carotid artery unstable plaques with 18F-fluorodeoxyglucose (FDG)-positron emission tomography (PET) imaging.[3,4] Molecular and functional imaging modalities to assess CVD with PET and others are rapidly

emerging, and, although their clinical application is still limited currently, they are expected to play a crucial role in the workup on CVD in the near future. In this issue of *PET Clinics*, we present a series of state-of-the-art articles regarding the application of multimodality functional imaging in CVD, primarily with PET, cardiac CT, and cardiac MRI.

Various PET applications in CVD are covered in detail, with an emphasis on FDG-PET/CT imaging. FDG remains the dominant radiopharmaceutical for oncologic PET applications, and we are just starting to realize the tremendous potential of FDG in evaluating various chronic inflammatory diseases and assessing disease status and response to therapy. Although myocardial perfusion with PET using rubidium and ammonia is becoming more prevalent, cardiac metabolic imaging with FDG to assess viability in combination with perfusion imaging remains an important application for PET in evaluating chronic ischemic heart disease and cardiac dysfunction. The underlying mechanism, imaging protocol, scan interpretation, and clinical significance of FDG-PET viability studies have been discussed in detail. Reviews of applications of FDG-PET in evaluating cardiac sarcoidosis, unstable atherosclerotic plaque in major arteries, and the more recent advances in myocardial scar mapping during ventricular tachycardia ablation appear timely,

PET Clin 6 (2011) xi–xii
doi:10.1016/j.cpet.2011.10.005

especially the latter since it could be the next frontier in cardiac electrophysiology.[5] A cardiologist's view about imaging in CVD brings an important clinical perspective to the needs and deficiencies with the current imaging approaches and highlights the modalities with the potential to have the most clinical impact on patient management. Lastly, reviews of nonnuclear imaging modalities in CVD including cardiac CT and cardiac MRI complete the issue with wide-ranging information on morphological evaluation and tissue characterization, especially with cardiac MRI, which can provide comprehensive cardiac evaluation in one setting and is covered in detail in this issue.

It is our belief that molecular and functional imaging in CVD predominantly with PET (with FDG and other novel PET probes) and other multimodality imaging techniques, including cardiac CT, cardiac MRI, and cardiac PET/MRI, will play an increasingly important role in the diagnosis and management of CVD. We hope that the readers are able to apply the knowledge from these articles in their clinical practice and research projects to combat the increasing menace of CVD. It has certainly been a pleasure for us to work on this important issue of *PET Clinics* with many of our colleagues; we really appreciate all their contributions and are proud of the final product.

Wengen Chen, MD, PhD
Department of Diagnostic Radiology
and Nuclear Medicine
University of Maryland School of Medicine
22 South Greene Street
Baltimore, MD 21201, USA

Amol M. Takalkar, MD, MS
Department of Radiology
Louisiana State University Health Sciences
Center–Shreveport, 1505 Kings Highway
Shreveport, LA 71103, USA

E-mail addresses:
wchen5@umm.edu (W. Chen)
atakalka@biomed.org (A.M. Takalkar)

REFERENCES

1. Lloyd-Jones D, Adams RJ, Brown TM, et al. Executive summary: heart disease and stroke statistics—2010 update: a report from the American Heart Association. Circulation 2010;121:948–54.
2. Chen W, Dilsizian V. (18)F-fluorodeoxyglucose PET imaging of coronary atherosclerosis and plaque inflammation. Curr Cardiol Rep 2010;12:179–84.
3. Wykrzykowska J, Lehman S, Williams G, et al. Imaging of inflamed and vulnerable plaque in coronary arteries with 18F-FDG PET/CT inpatients with suppression of myocardial uptake using a low-carbohydrate, high-fat preparation. J Nucl Med 2009;50:563–8.
4. Tawakol A, Migrino RQ, Bashian GG, et al. In vivo 18F-fluorodeoxyglucose positron emission tomography imaging provides a noninvasive measure of carotid plaque inflammation in patients. J Am Coll Cardiol 2006;48:1818–24.
5. Tian J, Smith MF, Chinnadurai P, et al. Clinical application of PET/CT fusion imaging for three-dimensional myocardial scar and left ventricular anatomy during ventricular tachycardia ablation. J Cardiovasc Electrophysiol 2009;20:597–604.

Role of FDG-PET in Evaluation of Myocardial Viability

Olga Molchanova-Cook, MD, PhD, Wengen Chen, MD, PhD*

KEYWORDS

- FDG-PET • Myocardial viability • Hibernating myocardium
- Revascularization

Heart failure is an enormous cardiovascular health problem worldwide. In the United States alone, 5 million patients suffer from symptomatic heart disease, and nearly 400,000 die each year. More than half a million patients are newly diagnosed with heart failure every year, and a much larger number of subjects may harbor asymptomatic ventricular dysfunctions. Coronary artery disease is an important contributor to the rise in the prevalence of heart failure and in associated mortality and morbidity. It is important that clinicians are able to predict evolution and progression of the disease so that appropriate preventive measures may be undertaken.

There is a complex interrelationship between mechanical cardiac function, myocardial perfusion, and metabolic and energy-consuming processes within the heart. In many patients with chronic coronary artery disease, impaired left ventricular function at rest arises in part from regions of ischemic or hibernating myocardium rather than scarred myocardium. Pathophysiologic paradigms have emerged that describe the relationship between myocardial perfusion and ventricular function pertaining to myocardial hibernation and stunning. In these paradigms, myocardial function is depressed but myocytes remain viable, and therefore left ventricular dysfunction can be reversed.

Evaluation of myocardial viability in heart failure allows for the prospective identification of patients with potentially reversible left ventricular dysfunction in whom prognosis may be favorably altered with coronary artery revascularization.

CARDIAC METABOLISM

One of the most important parts of cardiac metabolism involves conversion of energy substrates into the fuel for ATP production. ATP is then used to support myocardial contraction and to regulate ATP-dependent pumps in the cell membrane. For a given physiologic environment, the heart consumes the most efficient energy substrate. In the normally oxygenated heart in a fasting state, fatty acids account for most ATP production with glucose making only a small contribution to the ATP production, unless there is an insulin surge. During an acute increase in work load (eg, inotropic stimulation) the heart immediately mobilizes its glycogen reserve with transient increase in glycogen oxidation, to meet the need for additional energy by oxidation of carbohydrate substrates (glucose and lactate).

The breakdown of fatty acids in the mitochondria by β-oxidation is exquisitely sensitive to oxygen deprivation. Under anaerobic conditions, the myocytes compensate for loss of oxidative potential by shifting toward greater use of glucose to generate high energy phosphates, with simultaneous downregulation of mitochondrial oxidative metabolism and reduction of contractile function. Conversion of glucose via glucose-6-phosphate and pyruvate provides the source of acetyl-CoA, which is subsequently used in the tricarboxylic acid cycle for ATP production. For every 1 mol of glucose metabolized through glycolysis, 2 mol of ATP are generated (anaerobic condition).

The authors have nothing to disclose.
Department of Diagnostic Radiology and Nuclear Medicine, University of Maryland School of Medicine, 22 South Greene Street, Baltimore, MD 21201, USA
* Corresponding author.
E-mail address: wchen5@umm.edu

PET Clin 6 (2011) 383–391
doi:10.1016/j.cpet.2011.08.003

Because glycolysis can generate ATP under anaerobic conditions, glycolysis becomes an attractive alternate metabolic pathway for ATP generation in hypoperfused myocardium with a limited supply of oxygen. The metabolic switch of major energy substrate from fatty acids to glucose represents one of the earliest adaptive responses to myocardial ischemia (**Fig. 1**).

PHYSIOLOGY OF HIBERNATING MYOCARDIUM

The imbalance between oxygen supply, usually caused by reduced myocardial perfusion, and oxygen demand, determined primarily by the rate and force of myocardial contraction, is termed "ischemic myocardium." The phenomena of stunning, hibernation, and ischemic preconditioning represent different mechanisms of acute and chronic adaptation to a temporary or sustained reduction in coronary blood flow.[1]

Hibernating myocardium refers to resting left ventricular dysfunction caused by reduced coronary blood flow that can be partially or completely reversed by myocardial revascularization. Hibernating myocardium represents dysfunctional but viable myocardium most likely the result of extensive metabolic, structural, and functional remodeling in response to repetitive episodes of myocardial ischemia, termed "programmed cell survival." This process is thought to be partly associated with preferential metabolism of glucose and

increased glycogen content in the myocytes, simulating the fetal heart. Such changes have been attributed to a dedifferentiation process. Moreover, hibernating myocytes have been shown to reexpress contractile proteins that are specific to the fetal heart, such as α-smooth muscle cell actin. Recent studies on programmed cell survival and apoptosis support a direct link between metabolic pathways and cellular adaptation or maladaptation. It has been proposed that perhaps metabolic reprogramming of the ischemic myocardium initiates and sustains the functional and structural remodeling of hibernating myocardium.[2–5]

Myocardial hibernation is the most dramatic example of metabolic switch of energy substrates. Although the amount of energy produced by glycolysis may be adequate to maintain myocyte viability and preserve the electrochemical gradient across the cell membrane, it may not be sufficient to sustain contractile function. In hibernation, the adaptive response of the myocardium in the setting of prolonged resting hypoperfusion (reduced oxygen supply) is a reduction in myocardial contractile function (reduced oxygen demand), thereby preserving myocardial viability in the absence of clinically evident ischemia.

Although in acute ischemia there is a switch in energy substrate preference from fatty acids to glucose, metabolic gene expression in repetitive ischemia is not yet well described. In the heart the peroxisome proliferation-activated receptor α, a transcription factor that modulates fatty acid

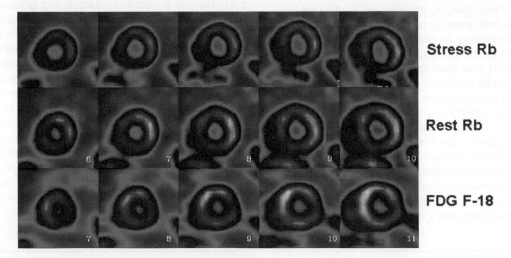

Apex ⟷ Base

Fig. 1. PET perfusion-metabolism imaging in a patient with critical stenosis of the right coronary artery. Stress myocardial perfusion rubidium-82 PET images show an area of decreased perfusion in the inferior and inferoseptal regions of the left ventricle, which appears to be reversible on rest rubidium images. FDG-PET images demonstrate relatively increased activity in the ischemic regions of the myocardium, compatible with metabolic switch of preferential energy substrate from fatty acids to glucose as an adaptive response to myocardial ischemia.

metabolism, regulates the substrate preference. In a mouse model of ischemic cardiomyopathy, the role of metabolic gene expression induced by repetitive ischemia was assessed. In response to repetitive ischemia, there was a reversible down-regulation of the genes that modulate fatty acid metabolism and myosin heavy chain isoforms in the heart. Overexpression of extracellular super-oxide dismutase, an endogenous antioxidant enzyme, in hearts exposed to repetitive ischemia failed to cause the decrease in metabolic and myosin isoform gene expression. When fatty acid metabolism in hearts exposed to repetitive ischemia was pharmacologically reactivated, there was worsening of contractile function, micro-infarctions, and triglyceride accumulation within cardiomyocytes. These findings suggest that downregulation of fatty acid metabolic gene expression in the hibernating myocardium is an adaptive mechanism. Furthermore, modulation of myocardial metabolism may provide a pharmaco-logic target for cardiac protection in repetitive ischemia.[6,7]

METHODS OF MYOCARDIAL VIABILITY EVALUATION

The most common definition of myocardial viability is the temporal improvement in contractile function of a dysfunctional myocardial region after restoration of blood flow. Requirements for cellular viability include sufficient myocardial blood flow, intact sarcolemmal membrane function, and preserved metabolic activity.

Myocardial blood flow has to be adequate to deliver substrate to the myocytes to be used in the metabolic process, and to remove the end products of the metabolic process. If regional blood flow is severely reduced or absent, then the metabolites and end products accumulate, causing inhibition of the enzymes of the metabolic pathway, depletion of high-energy phosphates, cell membrane disruption, and cell death. Thus, at either extreme of the range of blood flow, myocardial perfusion tracers provide information regarding myocardial viability. Perfusion can be evaluated by technetium-99m (Tc-99m) labeled radiotracers, thallium-201, or rubidium-82. However, in the regions in which the reduction in blood flow is of intermediate severity, perfusion information alone may be insufficient to determine viability, and additional data, such as metabolic indices, are necessary.[1]

Another requirement for cardiomyocyte viability is intact sarcolemmal membrane function to main-tain electrochemical gradients across the cell membrane. Because cell membrane integrity is highly dependent on preserved intracellular metabolic activity to generate high energy phos-phates, tracers that reflect sarcolemmal cation flux and perfusion, such as thallium-201 and rubidium-82, should parallel the viability informa-tion provided by markers of metabolic activity (eg, F18-fluorodexyglucose [FDG]). In the setting of reduced regional blood flow and function, tech-niques that assess intact cellular sarcolemmal function or metabolic processes provide unique insight into the presence or absence of myocardial viability.

The principle of using metabolic tracers for viability evaluation is based on the concept that viable myocytes in hypoperfused and dysfunc-tional regions are metabolically active, whereas scarred or fibrotic tissue is metabolically inactive.

FDG is a radioactive glucose analog used to image myocardial glucose use with PET. After intravenous injection, FDG is transported across the sarcolemma like glucose and is phosphory-lated by hexokinase to FDG-6-phosphate, which is impermeable to the sarcolemma. Once phos-phorylated, FDG is not metabolized further in the glycolytic pathway, fructose-pentose shunt, or glycogen synthesis. Because the dephosphoryla-tion rate of FDG in the myocytes is slow, essentially it becomes trapped in the myocardium, allowing adequate time to image regional glucose uptake. Preserved or increased myocardial glucose use in the regions of rest hypoperfusion) is consistent with viable myocardium. These are the funda-mental bases of FDG-PET imaging to assess myocardial glucose metabolism in the clinical setting.[8]

Myocardial FDG uptake is influenced by meta-bolic and hormonal milieu. In the fasting and aerobic conditions, fatty acids are the preferred source of myocardial energy production, with glucose accounting for 15% to 20% of the total energy supply. However, in the fed state, plasma insulin level increases, glucose metabolism is stimulated, and lipolysis is inhibited, resulting in reduced fatty acid delivery to the myocardium. The combined effects of insulin on these pro-cesses and the increased arterial glucose concen-tration associated with fed state result in preferred glucose use by the myocardium.[1] Preserved or increased myocardial glucose use in the regions of rest hypoperfusion is consistent with viable myocardium.

Viable myocardial regions also can be identified using thallium-201 scintigraphy. Thallium-201 has been used and investigated extensively for identi-fying myocardial viability and hibernation, and is the first radiotracer to be used for this purpose. The two most common protocols optimized for viability detection are rest-redistribution and stress-4-hour-redistribution-reinjection protocols. The rest-redistribution protocol assesses myocardial viability alone, whereas the stress-redistribution-reinjection protocol assesses myocardial ischemia and viability. On the thallium images, decrease in the left ventricular perfusion defect size from rest to redistribution represents hibernating but viable myocardium. When taking into consideration regions with reversible defects (ischemia) and success of revascularization (reexamining regional perfusion or vessel patency after revascularization), stress-redistribution-reinjection thallium imaging yields excellent positive and negative predictive accuracy for recovery of function after revascularization.[9,10]

Despite the excellent flow kinetics and biologic properties of thallium-201, the low-energy gamma ray emission and long half-life of thallium-201 are potential limitations, leading to attenuation of photons, particularly in patients with a large body habitus, and higher radiation exposure compared with Tc-99m–labeled perfusion tracers.

Nitrate-enhanced Tc-99m tracer studies involve acquisition of two sets of images: a rest image and a nitrate-enhanced image. Nitrates enhance collateral blood flow and radiotracer uptake in hypoperfused myocardial regions. Perfusion defect reversibility after nitrate administration is considered to be indicative of viability.[11,12]

New high-energy collimators for single-photon emission computed tomography (SPECT) cameras can also be used for imaging of positron-emitting tracers, such as F18-FDG. Differences between SPECT and PET technologies and between FDG and thallium tracers were examined in patients with chronic coronary artery disease to determine whether FDG-SPECT could be adopted for assessment of myocardial viability. Receiver-operating characteristics curves showed overall good concordance between SPECT and PET technologies and thallium and FDG tracers for assessing viability. However, in the subgroup of patients with left ventricular ejection fraction (LVEF) of 25% or less, thallium tended to underestimate myocardial viability. In a subgroup of regions with severe asynergy, there were considerably more thallium-FDG discordances in the inferior wall than elsewhere (73% vs 27%; $P<.001$), supporting attenuation of thallium as a potential explanation for the discordant observations. It was shown that FDG-SPECT significantly increases the sensitivity for detection of viable myocardium compared with thallium, and showed up to 88% of the sensitivity achievable by PET. However, in 27% of cases it falsely identified tissue as viable when it had been identified as nonviable by PET and thallium.[13]

PET has several technical advantages over gamma-technique SPECT, such as higher counting sensitivity, higher spatial resolution, routine use of more accurate attenuation correction, and absolute quantification of myocardial perfusion flow and metabolism.

Dobutamine echocardiography can be used for myocardial viability evaluation. Hibernating but viable myocardium is identified as regions of myocardium with abnormal resting systolic function but manifesting contractile reserve during dobutamine administration.[12,14]

Contrast-enhanced cardiac MR imaging has been successfully used for the assessment of scarred myocardium in chronic left ventricular dysfunction. While studying myocardial perfusion patterns in patients with acute and chronic myocardial infarction, increased signal intensity (greater T1 shortening after contrast) was observed in the infarcted, nonviable myocardium (~10 minutes after bolus injection of the contrast), and was termed "delayed enhancement." Reversibly injured myocardium did not exhibit increased contrast concentration or enhancement. The current technique involves rapid infusion of gadolinium chelate followed by a high-resolution cardiac-gated T1-weighted pulse sequence 5 to 30 minutes thereafter. If imaging is performed too early (<5 minutes after contrast infusion) or too late (>30 minutes after contrast infusion), it may result in underestimation or overestimation of infarct size. Because the contrast used is primarily an extracellular, interstitial agent, it has been hypothesized that it is the increased volume of distribution of the contrast molecules within the infarcted imaging voxel that is responsible for the greater shortening of the T1 relaxation time.[15] The accuracy of this technique has been validated by comparison with histopathology,[16] nuclear techniques,[17] and recovery of function (or lack thereof) after revascularization.[15]

A principal advantage of nuclear techniques (PET and SPECT) is the synergy that exists between the modality and underlying physiologic states being investigated, because the radiotracers used, by nature, reflect physiologic processes at the cellular level.

FDG-PET IMAGE QUALITY OPTIMIZATION AND STANDARDIZATION

The diagnostic quality of FDG imaging is critically dependent on many factors, such as hormonal milieu, substrate availability, and regional blood flow. This becomes particularly evident when studying patients with clinical or subclinical diabetes. Most clinical studies are performed after 50- to 75-g glucose loading with oral dextrose approximately 1 to 2 hours before the FDG injection. Although 90% of FDG images are of adequate-to-excellent diagnostic quality in nondiabetic patients, the quality of FDG images after glucose loading is less consistent in patients with clinical or subclinical diabetes mellitus. Because increase in plasma insulin levels after glucose loading may be attenuated in patients with diabetes mellitus, tissue lipolysis is not inhibited, and free fatty acid levels in the plasma remain high. Acquiring good quality FDG images in diabetics may be challenging. Standardization schemes used to optimize FDG image quality include intravenous insulin injections after glucose loading, hyperinsulinemic-euglycemic clamping, and use of a nicotinic acid derivative.

Intravenous bolus of regular insulin is clinically feasible and the most commonly used approach. Regular insulin is administered according to the plasma glucose level and a predetermined sliding scale. Plasma glucose level is assessed every 15 minutes with the administration of additional boluses of insulin, if necessary. The FDG dose is injected once the plasma glucose level is less than 140 mg/dL.

With hyperinsulinemic-euglycemic clamping, insulin and glucose are infused simultaneously to achieve a stable plasma insulin level of 100 to 120 IU/L and a normal plasma glucose level. The rate of glucose infusion (20% dextrose solution with potassium chloride) is adjusted intermittently based on measured glucose levels. Although it provides excellent image quality, the technique is rather tedious and impractical for routine clinical studies.

When using nicotinic acid derivative for image optimization, approximately 2 hours before the FDG dose injection, a single dose of nicotinic acid derivative is given orally followed by glucose loading. The resulting FDG image quality has been shown to be comparable with that of the clamp technique in the same patient population.[1]

ROLE OF FDG-PET MYOCARDIAL VIABILITY IN CLINICAL PRACTICE

LVEF is a major determinant of survival in patients with acute and chronic coronary artery disease. The Multicenter Postinfarction Trial showed curvilinear relationship between mortality rates in the first year after myocardial infarction and predischarge LVEF in patients with acute myocardial infarction, with the highest mortality rates observed in the patients with LVEF less than 20%. There was a dramatic decrease in mortality rates with increasing LVEF, which reached a plateau at the lowest mortality rate in patients with preserved left ventricular function (LVEF >50%).[18] This relationship has been demonstrated conclusively in virtually every study assessing patient outcome after myocardial infarction. The cumulative 4-year survival of medically treated Coronary Artery Surgery Study (CASS) registry patients with chronic stable coronary artery disease and normal (>50%) or mildly reduced (35%–49%) LVEF at rest was shown to be 92% and 83%, respectively. However, patients with moderate to severely reduced (<34%) left ventricular function had a significantly lower 4-year survival (58%) when treated with medical therapy alone.[19]

Among the CASS registry patients, short- and long-term surgical survival benefits were greatest in patients with the most severe left ventricular dysfunction. Among the patients with LVEF less than 25%, the 5-year survival rate was 62% with surgical treatment and 41% with medical treatment. The 1- and 2-year survival rates of surgically treated patients were 85% and 77%, comparing with 76% and 66% in the medically treated patients, respectively.[20]

Data from a metaanalysis of 3088 patients (mean LVEF 32%, followed for 25 ± 10 months) demonstrates that in patients with preserved myocardial viability the annual mortality rate was significantly lower in those who were treated with revascularization (3.2%) compared with those treated with medical therapy alone (16%). This represents a 79.6% decrease in annual mortality in patients with viable myocardium treated with revascularization (P<.0001). Moreover, there was a direct relationship between the severity of left ventricular dysfunction and the magnitude of benefit from revascularization among patients with myocardial viability (P<.001). In contrast, among patients without evidence of viable myocardium, there was no incremental benefit of revascularization over medical therapy. These data support the role of myocardial viability testing for management of patients with chronic left ventricular dysfunction and in guiding therapeutic decisions for revascularization.[21]

By definition, myocardial viability implies the temporal improvement in contractile function of a dysfunctional myocardial region after restoration of blood flow. Thus, evaluation of myocardial viability in patients with severely reduced left ventricular function provides for the prospective identification of patients with potentially reversible left ventricular dysfunction in whom prognosis may be favorably altered with coronary artery revascularization.[22]

Patients with severe left ventricular dysfunction who undergo revascularization can have a considerable risk of procedure-related morbidity and mortality. Identification of patients with the potential for improvement in LVEF and survival is needed to justify the higher risk of therapeutic intervention in these patients. With increased surgical expertise and improved intraoperative myocardial preservation techniques, combined with accurate prospective assessment of myocardial viability, surgical mortality rates will decrease further.

Hibernating myocardium represents dysfunctional but viable myocardium most likely the result of extensive cellular reprogramming caused by repetitive episodes of ischemia. It is considered an adaptive rather than an injurious response to chronic ischemia. One of the earliest adaptive responses to myocardial ischemia is a metabolic switch of major energy substrate from fatty acids to glucose. Because glucose transport and phosphorylation can be readily tracked by the uptake and retention of FDG, hibernating myocardium can be detected by enhanced FDG uptake in these regions on FDG-PET images.

Preserved or increased myocardial glucose use in the region of resting hypoperfusion is termed a "mismatch pattern." In **Fig. 2**, rest myocardial perfusion rubidium-82 PET images show severely reduced blood flow in the distal anterior, anteroseptal, and apical regions of the left ventricle, with preserved metabolism on the FDG images consistent with myocardial viability. These findings in the setting of heart failure symptoms secondary to ischemic left ventricular dysfunction portend good outcome after revascularization.

Reduced or absent myocardial glucose use in hypoperfused myocardial regions is termed a "match pattern." In **Fig. 3**, rest myocardial perfusion rubidium-82 PET images show severely reduced blood flow in the entire inferior region of the left ventricle. The same area shows absent myocardial metabolism on the FDG images. This is consistent with scarred myocardium.

In many patients with chronic coronary artery disease, impaired left ventricular function at rest arises in part from regions of ischemic or hibernating myocardium rather than scarred myocardium.[23] The application of described PET patterns in patients with chronic ischemic left ventricular dysfunction confers high positive and negative predictive accuracies for recovery of regional function after revascularization, with an overall accuracy between 80% and 90%.[24] However, clinically meaningful increases in global left ventricular function after revascularization are best attained if the extent of hibernating and stunned myocardium is 17% to 25% of the left ventricular mass or more.[25]

The prognostic significance of perfusion–metabolism mismatch pattern in ischemic cardiomyopathy has been shown in nonrandomized, retrospective studies with PET.[26,27] Patients with a perfusion–metabolism mismatch pattern who were treated surgically had lower ischemic event rates and fewer deaths compared with those treated with medical therapy. In contrast, patients with perfusion–metabolism match pattern displayed no such difference in outcomes between surgical and medical management. Moreover, the patients with myocardial viability (mismatch pattern) who underwent revascularization manifested a significant improvement in heart failure symptoms and exercise tolerance.[28,29]

The anatomic extent of perfusion–metabolism PET mismatch pattern (expressed as percent of the left ventricle) is proportional to the change in functional status after revascularization (expressed

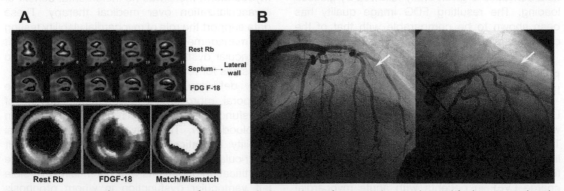

Fig. 2. PET imaging demonstrating perfusion-metabolism mismatch pattern in a patient with chronic total occlusion of the left anterior descending coronary artery (LAD) stent. (*A*) Rest myocardial perfusion rubidium-82 PET images show severely reduced blood flow in the distal anterior, anteroseptal, and apical regions of the left ventricle, with preserved metabolism on the F-18 FDG images consistent with myocardial viability. (*B*) Coronary angiogram shows total occlusion of the LAD stent (*arrows*). These findings in the setting of heart failure symptoms secondary to ischemic left ventricular dysfunction portend good outcome after revascularization.

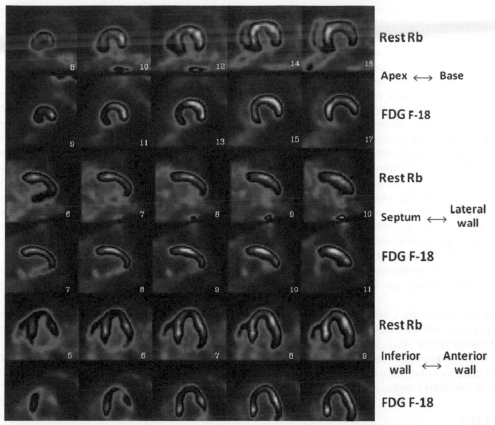

Rest Rb

Apex ⟷ Base

FDG F-18

Rest Rb

Septum ⟷ Lateral wall

FDG F-18

Rest Rb

Inferior wall ⟷ Anterior wall

FDG F-18

Fig. 3. PET imaging demonstrating perfusion-metabolism match pattern in a patient with total occlusion of the right coronary artery. Rest myocardial perfusion rubidium-82 PET images show severely reduced blood flow in the entire inferior region of the left ventricle. The same area shows absent myocardial metabolism on the F-18 FDG images. This is consistent with scarred myocardium.

as percent improvement from baseline) with the greatest improvement in heart failure symptoms achieved in patients with the largest mismatch defects on quantitative analysis of PET images. The receiver-operating characteristic curve for different anatomic extent of perfusion–metabolism mismatch to predict a change (at least one grade) in functional status after revascularization was calculated. When the extent of PET mismatch involves 18% or more of the left ventricular mass, the sensitivity for predicting a change in functional status after revascularization is 76% and the specificity is 78% (area under the fitted curve = 0.82).[28]

The determination of myocardial viability in patients with coronary artery disease and severe left ventricular dysfunction before referral for coronary revascularization affects clinical outcome with respect to both in-hospital mortality and 1-year survival rate. It was shown in a retrospective study that perioperative and postoperative event-free survival rate was significantly lower in patients who were referred to revascularization on the basis of clinical presentation and angiographic data but without viability testing, compared with those who were selected according to the extent of viable tissue determined by PET in addition to clinical presentation and angiographic data. After 12 months, the survival rates were 79% and 97%, respectively (P = .01).[29]

Irrespective of the imaging modality applied for evaluation of myocardial viability, the recovery of function after revascularization seems to be a continuum and is coupled to the ratio of viable to scarred myocardium within dysfunctional myocardial segments. It was demonstrated that the extent of infarction on cardiac magnetic resonance or percent thallium defect on SPECT correlate with decreasing likelihood of functional recovery after revascularization.[9,15]

Unfortunately, because structural changes in hibernating myocardium are chronic in nature and have developed over a prolonged period, some regions as shown viable by scintigraphic or echocardiographic techniques may be irreversible despite successful revascularization. In the multi-center Surgical Treatment for Ischemic Heart Failure trial substudy, the presence of viable myocardium was associated with a greater likelihood of survival in patients with coronary artery disease and left ventricular dysfunction (LVEF <35%) who were randomized to receive medical therapy plus coronary artery bypass grafting (CABG) versus receiving medical therapy alone. However, this relationship was not significant after adjustment for other prognostic baseline variables. SPECT, dobutamine echocardiography, or both were used to assess myocardial viability. These findings do not necessarily indicate that myocardial viability does not have pathophysiologic importance in patients with coronary artery disease and left ventricular dysfunction. Instead, it is likely that some of the other variables in the analysis (eg, left ventricular volumes, LVEF) are causally determined by the extent of viable myocardium.[30]

Medical therapy, like CABG, also has the potential to improve left ventricular function in patients with dysfunctional but viable myocardium.[31] These findings highlight the need for prospective studies to further clarify the role of cardiac imaging in clinical decision making.

SUMMARY

In many patients with chronic coronary artery disease, impaired left ventricular function at rest arises in part from regions of ischemic or hibernating myocardium rather than scarred myocardium. Evaluation of myocardial viability in heart failure allows for the prospective identification of patients with potentially reversible left ventricular dysfunction in whom prognosis may be favorably altered with coronary artery revascularization. Like CABG, medical therapy also has the potential to improve left ventricular function in patients with dysfunctional but viable myocardium. These findings highlight the need for prospective studies to further clarify the role of cardiac imaging in clinical decision making.

REFERENCES

1. Taegtmeyer H, Dilsizian V. Imaging cardiac metabolism. In: Narula J, Dilsizian V, editors. Atlas of nuclear cardiology. 3rd edition. Philadelphia: Current Medicine Group LLC; 2009. p. 182.

2. Depre C, Taegtmeyer H. Metabolic aspects of programmed cell survival and cell death in the heart. Cardiovasc Res 2000;45:538–48.

3. Kim HD, Kim DJ, Lee IJ, et al. Human fetal heart development after mid–term: morphometry and ultrastructural study. J Mol Cell Cardiol 1992;24: 949–65.

4. Taegtmeyer H, Sharma S, Goldman L, et al. Linking gene expression to function: metabolic flexibility in normal and diseased heart. Ann N Y Acad Sci 2004;1015:1–12.

5. Taegtmeyer H. Modulation of responses to myocardial ischemia: metabolic features of myocardial stunning, hibernation, and ischemic preconditioning. In: Dilsizian V, Armonk, editors. Myocardial viability: a clinical and scientific treatise. New York: Futura; 2000. p. 25–36.

6. Dewald O, Sharma S, Adrogue J, et al. Downregulation of peroxisome proliferator–activated receptor–alpha gene expression in a mouse model of ischemic cardiomyopathy is dependent on reactive oxygen species and prevents lipotoxicity. Circulation 2005;112:407–15.

7. Golfman LS, Wilson CR, Sharma S, et al. Activation of PPARgamma enhances myocardial glucose oxidation and improves contractile function in isolated working hearts of ZDF rats. Am J Physiol Endocrinol Metab 2005;289:E328–36.

8. Nguyen VT, Mossberg KA, Tewson TJ, et al. Temporal analysis of myocardial glucose metabolism by 2–[18F]fluoro–2–deoxy–D–glucose. Am J Physiol 1990;259:H1022–31.

9. Kitsiou AN, Srinivasan G, Quyyumi AA, et al. Stress–induced reversible and mild–to–moderate irreversible thallium defects: are they equally accurate for predicting recovery of regional left ventricular function after revascularization? Circulation 1998;98: 501–8.

10. Dilsizian V, Rocco TP, Freedman NM, et al. Enhanced detection of ischemic but viable myocardium by the reinjection of thallium after stress–redistribution imaging. N Engl J Med 1990;323:141–6.

11. Bisi G, Sciagra R, Santoro GM, et al. Rest technetium–99m sestamibi tomography in combination with short–term administration of nitrates: feasibility and reliability for prediction of postrevascularization outcome of asynergic territories. J Am Coll Cardiol 1994;24:1282–9.

12. Leoncini M, Marcucci G, Sciagra R, et al. Nitrate–enhanced gated technetium 99m sestamibi SPECT for evaluating regional wall motion at baseline and during low–dose dobutamine infusion in patients with chronic coronary artery disease and left ventricular dysfunction: comparison with two–dimensional echocardiography. J Nucl Cardiol 2000;7:426–31.

13. Srinivasan G, Kitsiou AN, Bacharach SL, et al. 18F–Fluorodeoxyglucose single photon emission computed tomography: can it replace PET and thallium SPECT for the assessment of myocardial viability? Circulation 1998;97:843–50.

14. Williams MJ, Odabashian J, Lauer MS, et al. Prognostic value of dobutamine echocardiography in

patients with left ventricular dysfunction. J Am Coll Cardiol 1990;27:192–9.

15. Kim RJ, Wu E, Rafael A, et al. The use of contrast–enhanced magnetic resonance imaging to identify reversible myocardial dysfunction. N Engl J Med 2000;343:1445–53.

16. Arnado LC, Gerber BI, Gupta SN, et al. Accurate and objective infarct sizing by contrast–enhanced magnetic resonance imaging in a canine myocardial infarction model. J Am Coll Cardiol 2004;44:2383–9.

17. Klein C, Nekolla SG, Bengel FM, et al. Assessment of myocardial viability with contrast–enhanced magnetic resonance imaging: comparison with positron emission tomography. Circulation 2002;105:162–7.

18. The Multicenter Postinfarction Research Group. Risk stratification and survival after myocardial infarction. N Engl J Med 1983;309:331–6.

19. Mock MB, Ringqvist I, Fisher LD, et al. Survival of medically treated patients in the coronary artery surgery study (CASS) registry. Circulation 1982;66:562–8.

20. Alderman EL, Fisher LD, Litwin P, et al. Results of coronary artery surgery in patients with poor left ventricular function (CASS). Circulation 1983;68:785–95.

21. Allman KC, Shaw LJ, Hachamovitch R, et al. Myocardial viability testing and impact of revascularization on prognosis in patients with coronary artery disease and left ventricular dysfunction: a meta–analysis. J Am Coll Cardiol 2002;39:1151–8.

22. Elefteriades JA, Tolis G Jr, Levi E, et al. Coronary artery bypass grafting in severe left ventricular dysfunction: excellent survival with improved ejection fraction and functional state. J Am Coll Cardiol 1993;22:1411–7.

23. Braunwald E, Rutherford JD. Reversible ischemic left ventricular dysfunction: evidence for the "hibernating myocardium". J Am Coll Cardiol 1986;8:1467–70.

24. Tillisch JH, Brunken R, Marshall R, et al. Reversibility of cardiac wall motion abnormalities predicted by positron tomography. N Engl J Med 1986;314:884–8.

25. Dilsizian V, Arrighi JA. Myocardial viability in chronic coronary artery disease: perfusion, metabolism and contractile reserve. In: Gerson MC, editor. Cardiac nuclear medicine. 3rd edition. New York: McGraw–Hill; 1996. p. 143–91.

26. Eltzman D, Al–Aouar Z, Kanter HL, et al. Clinical outcome of patients with advanced coronary artery disease after viability studies with positron emission tomography. J Am Coll Cardiol 1992;20:559–65.

27. DiCarli MF, Davidson M, Little R, et al. Value of metabolic imaging with positron emission tomography for evaluating prognosis in patients with coronary artery disease and left ventricular dysfunction. Am J Cardiol 1994;73:527–33.

28. DiCarli MF, Asgarzadie F, Schebert HR, et al. Quantitative relation between myocardial viability and improvement in heart failure symptoms after revascularization in patient with ischemia cardiomyopathy. Circulation 1995;92:3436–44.

29. Haas F, Haehnel CJ, Picker W, et al. Preoperative positron emission tomography viability assessment and perioperative and postoperative risk in patients with advanced ischemic heart disease. J Am Cardiol 1997;30:1693–700.

30. Bonow RO, Maurer G, Lee KL, et al. Myocardial viability and survival in ischemic left ventricular dysfunction. N Engl J Med 2011;364:1617–25.

31. Cleland JG, Pennell DJ, Ray SG, et al. Myocardial viability as a determinant of the ejection fraction response to carvedilol in patients with heart failure (CHRISTMAS trial): randomized controlled trial. Lancet 2003;362:14–21.

Clinical Application of FDG-PET Imaging for Three-Dimensional Myocardial Scar and Left Ventricular Anatomy During Ventricular Tachycardia Ablation

Jing Tian, MD, PhD[a],*, Mark F. Smith, PhD[b],
Timm Dickfeld, MD, PhD[a]

KEYWORDS

- ^{18}F-Fluorodeoxyglucose PET • Myocardial scar
- Ventricular tachycardia ablation

INTRODUCTION

Ventricular tachycardia (VT) ablation is the next frontier in electrophysiology (EP). An increasing number of patients presenting with frequent and appropriate implantable cardioverter-defibrillator (ICD) firings require VT ablation despite optimal medical therapy.[1–5] Anatomically based substrate modification strategies have to be used in greater than 85% of these patients because of hemodynamic intolerance of the VT.[2] These approaches consist of linear ablation lines placed across and along the myocardial scar and its border zone to interrupt conducting channels of surviving myocardium.[2,6,7] Current clinical practice in VT ablation based on voltage mapping is limited by the inability to sufficiently characterize the myocardial substrate, such as scar, which represents the target of these ablations. In addition, suboptimal

catheter contact can result in falsely low voltage measurements. Scar characterization using PET imaging has been clinically established, extensively validated,[8,9] and its prognostic value has been demonstrated for cardiac interventions and cardiac surgery.[10,11] PET, magnetic resonance (MR) imaging, and x-ray computed tomography (CT) have been used retrospectively characterize as well as prospectively to guide VT ablation sites based on metabolic and anatomic scar characteristics.[12–18] Because of the relatively recent clinical application of 3-dimensional (3D) image integration using PET and other imaging modalities to guide VT ablation, there are no established image reconstruction/integration strategies or standard imaging criteria to define scar substrates. The relationships among scar substrates reconstructed from different modalities in the same patients and their relationships with the voltage map are still uncertain. In

The authors have nothing to disclose.
[a] Division of Cardiology, University of Maryland School of Medicine, 22 South Greene Street, Baltimore, MD 21201, USA
[b] Department of Diagnostic Radiology and Nuclear Medicine, University of Maryland School of Medicine, 22 South Greene Street, Baltimore, MD 21201, USA
* Corresponding author.
E-mail address: jtian@cdc.gov

PET Clin 6 (2011) 393–402
doi:10.1016/j.cpet.2011.08.005
1556-8598/11/$ – see front matter Published by Elsevier Inc.

this article, the authors review the mechanism of VT and scar characterization, different PET imaging reconstruction and integration methods, the comparison of 3D PET reconstructed scar and voltage scar, the comparison of quantitative PET intensities with voltage values in segmental analyses, and 3D scar reconstruction of other imaging modalities (MR imaging, CT) and their advantages/disadvantages compared with PET.

MECHANISM OF REENTRANT VENTRICULAR TACHYCARDIA

Myocardial scars are present in most patients with ischemic and nonischemic cardiomyopathy, and usually act as the substrate for reentrant VT.[5] According to pathologic findings, rather than being homogeneous tissue, cardiac scars often contain many channels of surviving myocardium, which enable electricity to enter, traverse, and exit the scar via different connections within this network and form a reentry loop maintaining reentrant VT (**Fig. 1**).[19,20] Cauterizing the myocardial channels along the scar border to interrupt those loops and clinical VT, therefore, is the aim of most reentrant VT ablations.

Because of hemodynamic intolerance as well as preexisting alternative channels and exit sites, an approach targeting single VT channels identified by their electrical characteristics will not be applicable for most patients.[2] A substrate-guided ablation approach is frequently conducted to treat such arrhythmias and involves the placement of linear ablation lesions along the scar border to interrupt as many channels as possible. These treatment strategies are the most commonly used and accepted ones.[2,21]

CURRENT GOLD STANDARD OF VOLTAGE MAPPING AND ITS LIMITATIONS

A detailed anatomic knowledge of scar location and its exact border is necessary to accurately place curative ablation lines. 3D mapping systems are currently used to create a voltage map of the left ventricle to obtain such anatomic information and is currently the gold standard.[2,21] The amplitude of endocardial voltages is measured and recorded in real time by a roving mapping catheter moved along the endocardial left ventricular (LV) surface.[21,22] The standard clinical voltage criteria include scar (<0.5 mV), border zone (0.5–1.5 mV), and healthy myocardium (>1.5 mV) (**Fig. 2**).[2] The border zone is the transition area between scar and healthy myocardium, and serves as the target for VT ablations.

However, voltage mapping has several important limitations. First, endocardial voltage is limited in distinguishing between nonviable and damaged

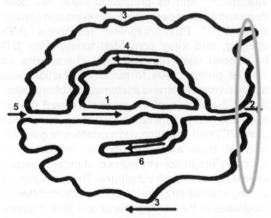

Fig. 1. Scar reentry. Myocardial scar displays a network of surviving myocardial channels. Reentry: During VT, the electrical wavefront quickly advances through normal myocardium around scar (**3**) and enters into the scar at the entry site (**5**). It slowly traverses the scar along surviving myocardial channels (**1**, **4**, and **6**) and exits the scar (**2**), which initiates the next cycle of conduction through normal myocardium to the entry site (**5**), establishing a reentry loop, maintaining VT. A continuous ablation line along the scar border (substrate, *green ellipsoid*) will interrupt the exit site and terminate the VT.

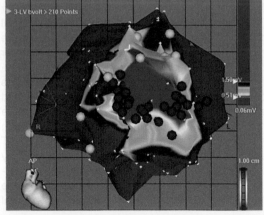

Fig. 2. Example of a voltage map. Red area represents scar with voltage values lower than 0.5 mV. Purple area represents healthy tissue with voltage values higher than 1.5 mV. Rainbow color in between represents the border zone area with voltage value higher than 0.5 mV but lower than 1. (*From* Tian J, Smith MF, Chinnadurai P, et al. Clinical application of PET/CT fusion imaging for three-dimensional myocardial scar and left ventricular anatomy during ventricular tachycardia ablation. J Cardiovasc Electrophysiol 2009;20:601; with permission.)

but viable myocardium, which can serve as a VT channel. Second, a single endocardial voltage measurement cannot differentiate between endocardial and epicardial scar components. Third, suboptimal catheter contact can result in falsely low voltage measurements, leading to an overestimation of ventricular scar and unnecessary ablation lesions. Fourth, the limited spatial resolution of the catheter tip of 5 to 15 mm and the mapping density of the voltage map can make it difficult to detect isolated scar areas or small patches of surviving myocardium that could represent viable VT channels. Finally, detailed voltage mapping is quite time consuming, which increases procedure length and complication rates. As a result, despite a procedure time of frequently longer than 5 hours, VTs can be eliminated with long-term success rates of only 53%.[23] Some of these limitations are currently being addressed by integrating preprocedural scar imaging into the VT ablation procedures.

PET IMAGING CHARACTERIZATION OF MYOCARDIAL SCAR

Recent advances in cardiac imaging have produced new tools for scar imaging and have provided the electrophysiologist with additional morphologic and metabolic definitions of myocardial scar. These techniques may be able to overcome some of the aforementioned limitations. The use of PET imaging to detect and characterize myocardial scar has been clinically established and extensively validated.[8,9] The combination of perfusion and metabolic PET imaging allowed a completely novel approach to assess the myocardial scar, enabling reentrant VT. It has been repeatedly validated for evaluation of: (1) nonviable myocardium; (2) diseased, but viable myocardium; and (3) normal cardiac tissue with results analogous to those derived from voltage maps. Thus it has successfully guided interventional and surgical revascularization strategies.[24,25]

SEGMENTAL ANALYSES TO COMPARE PET UPTAKE AND VOLTAGE MAP

At the University of Maryland, Rb-82 chloride perfusion and F-18 fluorodeoxyglucose (FDG) metabolic viability PET images have been analyzed using PMOD software (PMOD Technologies, Adliswil, Switzerland) using a 17-segment LV model.[26] PET signal intensities have been compared among segments of different voltage categories to discriminate them and further predict the presence of abnormal voltage segments. This information was used to guide the voltage mapping/ablation procedures.[27,28]

Segmental analysis was used in a recently published study that prospectively reviewed a cohort of 10 patients undergoing VT ablation and PET imaging. PET signal intensities of each segment were computed as a percentage of the maximum segment activity of the complete map for the individual perfusion and metabolic activity. The Rb-82 perfusion PET segments with peak uptake were considered normal myocardium, and the corresponding viability uptake value from the same FDG segment was used as 100% to normalize the FDG-PET data set. Voltage-defined scar and normal myocardium had perfusion-normalized FDG uptakes of 40% ± 13% and 89% ± 30%, respectively ($P<.05$).[14]

As a further step from the aforementioned study, the research group retrospectively reviewed a cohort of 13 patients with ischemic cardiomyopathy that underwent ^{82}Rb/^{18}F-FDG-PET imaging before VT ablation. The investigators compared FDG-PET metabolic activities among voltage scar, border zone, and normal myocardium segments. Voltage segments were defined by the standard clinical criteria of scar (<0.5 mV), border zone (0.5–1.5 mV), and normal myocardium (>1.5 mV). A 68-segment model developed by dividing each of the 17 segments of the American Heart Association model into 4 equally sized subregions was used to compare perfusion-normalized FDG uptakes among homogeneous (n = 327, 37%), voltage scar (n = 18, 2.2%), border zone (n = 15, 1.8%), and normal segments (n = 294, 35.3%). It confirmed that FDG uptakes differed significantly between scar and normal segments ($P<.05$), as well as between border zone and normal ($P<.05$) segments.[27]

In addition, the investigators also classified PET activities among this cohort into different categories, namely severe match (SMA, Rb <50%, FDG-Rb <10%), severe mismatch (SMI [hibernating], Rb <50%, FDG-Rb >10%), mild match (MMA, 50%<Rb<70%, FDG-Rb <10%), mild mismatch (MMI, 50%<Rb<70%, FDG-Rb >10%), and healthy (H, Rb >70%, FDG-Rb >10%). Voltage values were significantly different between healthy and individual nonhealthy segments (SMA, SMI, MMA, MMI, $P<.05$). Using 0.5 mV as the cutoff value to define scar myocardium, receiver operating characteristic (ROC) areas for Rb, FDG, and FDG-Rb were 0.75 ± 0.04, 0.67 ± 0.04, and 0.53 ± 0.05, respectively. Hibernating (SMI) myocardium segments have voltage features of scar (43%, n = 6), border zone (14%, n = 2), and normal (43%, n = 6).[28]

The aforementioned results indicated that perfusion-normalized FDG-PET imaging can provide quantitative measurement of the myocardium viability that enables the preprocedural determination of the electrophysiology voltage map and facilitates the actual mapping process. Polar plots of the FDG-PET can provide the preprocedural impressions of the voltage maps that will assist physicians in the procedures.

3D PET SCAR RECONSTRUCTION AND INTEGRATION METHODS

Preclinical image integration modules have been developed by different research centers to enable widespread, clinical use of image-reconstructed 3D scar maps to guide VT ablations. 3D metabolic scar maps were created to accurately display endocardial and epicardial surfaces, and could be successfully integrated with voltage maps.[13,14,29] These reconstructions are more direct than the 2-dimensional polar plots in terms of providing the preprocedural scar information, and could better assist the electrophysiological mapping.

The first attempt of 3D PET scar reconstruction was conducted by Dickfeld's group in 2005,[29] whereby PET images from a cohort of 10 patients were converted into DICOM3 format to allow recognition by the proprietary CartoMERGE software (Biosense Webster, Diamond Bar, CA). The investigators adjusted the upper and lower thresholds to color-code LV myocardium using the CartoMERGE image-processing tool. Viable

myocardium was defined by a board-certified nuclear cardiologist on the raw data set using 50% of the maximum value as the metabolic activity cutoff. The 3D cardiac model was extracted using the CartoMERGE software. This scar reconstruction strategy was also used in another article published later by Natale's group.[13]

Because the current version of CartoMERGE only allows a binary display (absent or present voxel), the myocardial scar had to be displayed as absent myocardium (ie, hole in the wall) in the aforementioned 3D scar reconstruction approach (**Fig. 3**). Although this approach can accurately reflect the location and size of the myocardial scar and border zone as assessed by the reading of a nuclear cardiologist, there can be registration errors between the 3D LV myocardium/scar and 3D voltage map.

In research published recently by Tian and colleagues,[14] DICOM-formatted FDG-PET images were postprocessed using MATLAB 7.6.0 (The Mathworks Inc, Natick, MA). FDG-derived myocardium and FDG-derived scar were coregistered with the CT data set to provide more anatomic detail and facilitate a more accurate registration with the electroanatomic voltage map. The myocardium from the PET images was automatically segmented using an algorithm based on level-set segmentation that uses implicit myocardial shape priors.[14] The segmented myocardium displayed both epicardial and endocardial surfaces (**Fig. 4**).

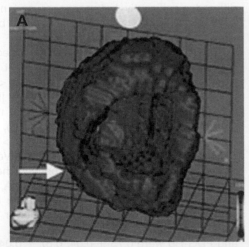 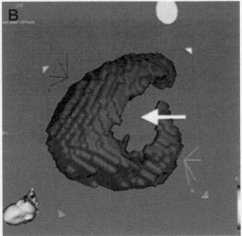

Fig. 3. Volume reconstruction of PET-derived 3-dimensional (3D) scar map in a clinical mapping system. The left ventricle is observed as an ocher-colored reconstruction from a basal orientation as indicated by the cardiac icon in the lower left corner (*A*). Three-dimensional reconstruction allows the visualization of the epicardium and also the endocardium, which can be visualized through the mitral valve plane. A basal, left lateral wall defect is seen as a hole in the reconstruction, signifying myocardial scar (*white arrow, A*). A left lateral view allows the visualization of the epicardium with an obvious wall defect caused by the myocardial scarring (*white arrow, B*). (*From* Dickfeld T, Lei P, Dilsizian V, et al. Integration of three-dimensional scar maps for ventricular tachycardia ablation using positron emission tomography/computed tomography (PET/CT). JACC Imaging 2008;1:77; with permission.)

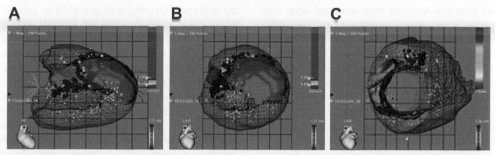

Fig. 4. Fusion of 3D LV anatomy and 3D scar reconstruction. The LV reconstruction is seen as a black mesh from anteroposterior (*A*), left anterior oblique (LAO) (*B*), and LAO cross-sectional (*C*) views allowing visualization of endocardium and epicardium surfaces. Areas in solid brown color represent myocardial scar embedded in the LV anatomy. Endocardial and epicardial scar surfaces can be visualized within the LV myocardium. (*From* Tian J, Smith MF, Chinnadurai P, et al. Clinical application of PET/CT fusion imaging for three-dimensional myocardial scar and left ventricular anatomy during ventricular tachycardia ablation. J Cardiovasc Electrophysiol 2009;20:600; with permission.)

The size and extent of the metabolic scar were qualitatively assessed by identifying the metabolic activity threshold that best represented the clinical scars. Multiple scar reconstructions were segmented from the FDG-PET myocardium using different thresholds ranging from 26% to 50% of the 100% FDG-PET value in 2% increments to cover the most clinically relevant metabolic range. A qualitative comparison was performed to determine which of the 13 threshold reconstructions best matched the voltage scar after the scar reconstructions were imported into CartoMERGE (Biosense Webster, Tirat Carmel, Israel).

The simultaneous 3D display of the LV anatomy and embedded myocardial scar as well as 3D scars constructed using different thresholds enabled the identification of not only myocardial scar but also myocardium with more preserved, but still abnormal, metabolic activity, which correlated with the voltage-defined border zone (**Fig. 5**). The border zone plays a critical role in VT ablation because greater than two-thirds of successful VT ablation sites are located within the border zone of myocardial scar.[7] This resulted in an immediate anatomy/substrate display, which is otherwise only available after a detailed endocardial voltage mapping. During the ablation, it allowed the electrophysiologist to focus on areas of likely myocardial scar and identify low-voltage recordings in areas of normal metabolism caused by suboptimal catheter contact.

COMPARISON OF 3D-RECONSTRUCTED PET SCAR AND VOLTAGE

Comparisons of 3D-reconstructed PET scar maps and their corresponding voltage maps showed good correlations. Dickfeld and colleagues[29]

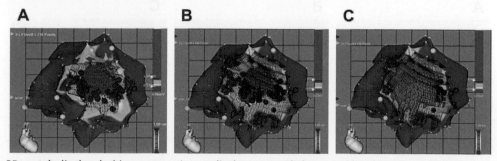

Fig. 5. 3D metabolic threshold reconstruction to display myocardial scar and border zone. Correlation of voltage map-defined scar with predefined metabolic threshold reconstructed scar (mesh, *A*). Increasing the metabolic threshold allows the identification of scar and additional metabolically abnormal myocardium that represents the voltage-defined border zone (mesh, *B*). The difference between metabolically defined scar as shown in B (represented by solid ocher 3D reconstruction) and metabolically abnormal myocardium as shown in C (represented by mesh) identifies voltage-defined border zone (*C*). (*From* Tian J, Smith MF, Chinnadurai P, et al. Clinical application of PET/CT fusion imaging for three-dimensional myocardial scar and left ventricular anatomy during ventricular tachycardia ablation. J Cardiovasc Electrophysiol 2009;20:601; with permission.)

reported that the voltage map–defined scar size and border zone demonstrated an overall good correlation with 3D scar map in patients with endocardially detected scar ($r = 0.86$, $r = 0.87$, respectively; $P<.05$). In these patients, 89% of the scar voltage map points (<0.5 mV) were within the metabolic scar area, with an additional 8% being within an adjacent 1- to 1.5-cm border zone. Voltage measurements within the PET-defined scar area demonstrated a voltage amplitude of only 0.3 ± 0.12 mV compared with 7.9 ± 5.4 mV in the area with normal metabolic activity ($P<.001$).

In the study by Tian and colleagues,[14] scar location and shape correlated well between the voltage map and the 3D FDG scar at the reconstruction threshold of 40% and the scar and border zone area at the reconstruction threshold of 46% (see **Fig. 5**). Simultaneous display of both reconstructions allowed the preprocedural display of scar and border zone area, and was used to provide supplemental metabolic data for the delineation of the linear ablation strategy. Fourteen segments out of 15 (93.3%) of the 3D metabolic scar-only segments matched with those in the voltage map. Fifteen segments out of 17 (88.2%) metabolic partial scar segments matched with those in the voltage map. In the article by Fahmy and colleagues,[13] instead of using different FDG thresholds for scar reconstructions, the voltage map settings were manually altered to fill the FDG-defined scar area. The investigators demonstrated that the best fit of the voltage-based scar with the PET scar was found at a threshold of 0.9 ± 0.15 mV for the patient cohort.

An additional value of 3D PET scar reconstructions is that integrated scar maps can provide additional scar characteristics that are not detectable by voltage mapping and are able to predict nontransmural scar in spite of normal endocardial voltage recordings. The study by Dickfeld and colleagues[29] indicated that PET provided a supplementary and sensitive way of assessing viable myocardium given the metabolic definition of cell survival. In the 3D scar maps for two patients with inferior infarctions, there were channels of viable myocardium in the scar areas, whose location matched with the successful ablation sites. In another patient with a lateral scar, there was a channel of viable myocardium crossing the scar, with all of the voltage mapping points less than 0.5 mV in the area. The mismatch between 3D PET scar reconstructions and their voltage recordings might represent endocardial scar indicated by low-voltage recordings in the scar area, but with significant epicardial or mid-myocardial surviving tissue that can be detected with PET (**Fig. 6**). Also in the same article, the investigators reported an example of PET helping to detect nontransmural epicardial scarring, whereby endocardial voltage mapping shows normal voltage recordings. Therefore, this technique may assist in planning the ablation strategies (**Fig. 7**).

3D SCAR RECONSTRUCTION OF OTHER IMAGING MODALITIES (MR IMAGING, CT) AND THEIR ADVANTAGES/DISADVANTAGES COMPARED WITH PET
Cardiac CT

Although FDG-PET provides a metabolic characterization of the myocardial scar and its border zone, the clinical spatial resolution of 6 to 8 mm and its restricted availability in cardiology practices limit its applicability. The recent technological

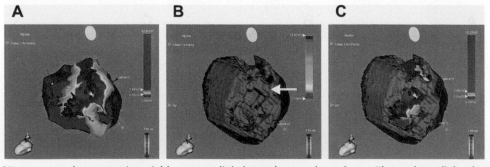

Fig. 6. 3D scar map demonstrating viable myocardial channel across lateral scar. The endocardial voltage map demonstrates an area of continuous lateral scar as defined by classical voltage criteria (*red area*) with adjacent yellow-to-blue border zone (*A*). The PET-derived 3D scar map in a corresponding view confirms a lateral scar (hole) but demonstrates a bridge of viable myocardium crossing the presumed scar area (*white arrow, B*). After registration of voltage map and 3D PET scar map, a bridge of metabolically alive tissue can be seen after successful registration traversing in the middle of the presumed voltage-defined myocardial scar (*red, C*). (*From* Dickfeld T, Lei P, Dilsizian V, et al. Integration of three-dimensional scar maps for ventricular tachycardia ablation using positron emission tomography/computed tomography (PET/CT). JACC Imaging 2008;1:80; with permission.)

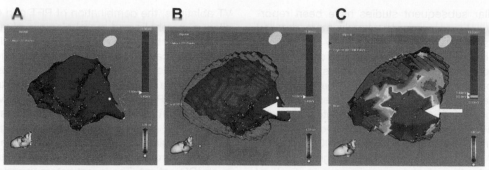

Fig. 7. 3D scar map displaying epicardial scar. The endocardial voltage map was unable to detect myocardial scar, and all wall segments revealed voltage of more than 1.5 mV (*left lateral view, A*). However, 3D PET scar map (ocher shell) reveals a large inferobasal lateral wall defect signifying myocardial scar, which was consistent with the exit site of the presenting ventricular tachycardia (*white arrow, B*). An epicardial voltage map finally confirmed a large, nontransmural scar (*red area*, 0.5 mV) in the inferobasal lateral location (*white arrow, C*). Registration of the epicardial voltage map and 3D PET scar map demonstrate good correlation between the epicardial voltage-defined scar and the PET-defined scar. (*From* Dickfeld T, Lei P, Dilsizian V, et al. Integration of three-dimensional scar maps for ventricular tachycardia ablation using positron emission tomography/computed tomography (PET/CT). JACC Imaging 2008;1:81; with permission.)

advances of contrast-enhanced computed tomography (CE-CT) enable submillimeter spatial resolution combined with acquisition times of 0.4 seconds or less, which makes detailed anatomic and dynamic characterization of global and regional myocardial function possible.[30–32]

The recent study by Tian and colleagues[33] is the first one to assess a comprehensive three-modality characterization (anatomic, dynamic, and perfusion) of LV scar from a single CE-CT scan, and demonstrates the ability to integrate this information into clinical mapping systems to guide VT ablation. Segmental anatomic (end-systolic/diastolic wall thickness [ESWT/EDST]), dynamic (wall thickening [WT] and wall motion), and perfusion (hypoenhancement) analyses indicated that abnormal anatomic, dynamic, and perfusion data correlated well with abnormal (<1.5 mV) endocardial voltages ($r = 0.77$). 3D reconstruction integrated into the clinical mapping system (registration accuracy: 3.31 ± 0.52 mm) allowed the prediction of homogeneous abnormal voltage (<1.5 mV) in 81.7% of analyzed segments, and correctly displayed transmural extent and intramural scar location. CT hypoperfusion correlated best with scar and border zone areas, and encompassed curative ablations in 82% of the cases.

Despite the aforementioned advantages, CE-CT still has several disadvantages that limit its usage. Because most of the patients undergoing VT ablation have an ICD installed, the presence of ICDs resulted in mild to moderate metal artifacts on CE-CT images, which could affect the quality of high-resolution data sets. In addition, nephrotoxic effects of CT contrast material are a significant concern,

especially because many cardiomyopathy/ICD patients present with underlying renal dysfunction.

Cardiac MR

Delayed-enhanced (DE) MR imaging is able to accurately characterize the location and transmural extent of myocardial scar.[34,35] Because of the different wash-in and wash-out kinetics, gadolinium is found in an increased concentration up to 20 minutes after injection in areas of myocardial necrosis/fibrosis, and imaged scar size correlates well with the histologic preparations.[36]

Codreanu and colleagues[16] reconstructed DE-MR images into 3D format and compared these reconstructions with the voltage map from the same patient to collect additional scar information. They found that MR imaging–reconstructed infarct surfaces best correlated to voltage-defined infarct areas defined by a cutoff value of less than 1.5 mV ($r^2 = 0.82$, $P<.0001$). When using the 1.5-mV cutoff, a mismatch of 20% in infarct surface measurement was observed in 4 of 12 scar areas (33%), with the presence of scar zones not confirmed on MR imaging views in 3 cases and underestimation of the infarct surface in the fourth. The investigators explained that mismatch typically occurred in regions (basal LV septum and posterior wall) where achievement of catheter stability and a good wall contact are technically challenging via the transaortic approach. As a consequence, a lower density of recorded points and/or acquisition of erroneous electrogram signals would result in a wrong definition of scar contours.

Similar subsequent studies have been reported by Bogun's group[17] wherein more detailed information was provided, especially the relationship between DE-MR imaging scar reconstructions and the characteristics of critical electrophysiological signals. In these studies the endocardial size of the scar, as assessed by DE-MR imaging (26 ± 34 cm²), correlated well with the endocardial scar size as defined by voltage mapping (<1.0 mV: $R = 0.96$; $P<.0001$, and <1.5 mV: $R = 0.94$; $P<.0001$). After integration of the scar into the electroanatomic map, activation/entrainment and/or pace mapping confirmed that the critical area for ventricular arrhythmias was confined to endocardial scar tissue in 7 of 14 patients (50%) with delayed enhancement. Epicardial mapping and ablation identified critical components of VT confined to epicardial scar in 2 of 14 patients (14%) with delayed enhancement. In 5 of 14 patients (36%) with delayed enhancement, scar was predominantly located intramurally and an ablation procedure was ineffective. Infarct depth correlated well with electrogram characteristics. Based on DE-MR imaging, all of the critical electrogram sites in the peripheral infarction zone were in an area of transmural infarct, with an MR imaging signal in its endocardial location slightly lower than the 3 standard deviation cutoff defining the core infarct zone.

Dickfeld and colleagues[37] have also reported that bipolar and unipolar voltages of 1.49 mV and 4.46 mV are the cutoff values that best differentiate the presence of endocardial MR imaging scar. Alive endocardium of greater than 2 mm resulted in greater than 1.5 mV voltage recordings despite up to 63% of transmural mid-myocardial scar being successfully ablated with MR imaging guidance.

Despite the detailed information of scar imaging and the relationship between scar zones/scar transmuralities and the electrophysiological characteristics provided by DE-MR imaging, DE-MR imaging has multiple limitations that prevent its widespread usage. First, the presence of an ICD still presents a contraindication in the majority of patients undergoing VT ablation.[38] Metal artifacts created by the ICD significantly affect the image quality, which makes accurate scar assessment impossible. In addition, the development of nephrogenic systemic fibrosis after gadolinium administration in patients with renal insufficiency has been recently reported.[39]

FUSION OR MULTIMODALITY IMAGING

The fusion of multiple imaging modalities will allow a more comprehensive scar characterization. For VT ablations, the combination of PET and CT will allow a metabolic and morphologic evaluation of the scar, its border zone, and the remaining left ventricular cavity. In the research by Dickfeld, Tian, and Natale, CT data have been used to help facilitate image orientations and registrations between 3D PET scar reconstructions and voltage maps. Recently, Tian and colleagues[15] reported a case with multimodality fusion imaging using DE-MR imaging, CT, PET, and real-time intracardiac echocardiography (ICE) to guide VT ablation in an ICD patient. The investigators reported that 20% to 30% of the DE-MR imaging scar with less than 25% transmurality in this patient was not detected by voltage mapping or PET. Those DE-MR imaging scar areas with abnormal voltage recordings/PET signals were consistent with greater than 25% to 50% transmurality. The investigators gave a possible explanation of this scar mismatch that the MR imaging could be more sensitive than the PET/voltage map in detecting scar. A thin layer of endocardial scar or isolated mid-myocardial/epicardial scar may not be detected by PET/voltage mapping. Tian and colleagues are investigating more detailed relationships among PET, DE-MR imaging, and voltage-defined scar areas for a patient cohort to facilitate the VT ablation guidance.

SUMMARY

PET imaging to detect and characterize myocardial scar has been applied to cardiac electrophysiology. Quantitative measurements of perfusion-normalized FDG-PET viability information as well as 3D PET scar reconstructions that integrate into voltage maps can provide preprocedural determination of the electrophysiology voltage map and predict nontransmural scar. This determination will facilitate the actual mapping process. Scar substrate information obtained before ablation procedures can shorten procedure length, increase insights into the reentrant VT substrate, and potentially optimize ablation results. Cardiac MR imaging and CT imaging, each with their own advantages and disadvantages, have been applied to cardiac electrophysiology. A combination of the aforementioned imaging modalities or multimodality fusion imaging will allow a more comprehensive scar characterization and provide important additional preprocedural information for reentrant VT ablation.

REFERENCES

1. Kadish A, Dyer A, Daubert JP, et al. Prophylactic defibrillator implantation in patients with nonischemic

dilated cardiomyopathy. N Engl J Med 2004;350: 2151–8.

2. Marchlinski FE, Callans DJ, Gottlieb CD, et al. Linear ablation lesions for control of unmappable ventricular tachycardia in patients with ischemic and nonischemic cardiomyopathy. Circulation 2000;101: 1288–96.

3. Moss AJ, Zareba W, Hall WJ, et al. Prophylactic implantation of a defibrillator in patients with myocardial infarction and reduced ejection fraction. N Engl J Med 2002;346:877–83.

4. Soejima K, Suzuki M, Maisel WH, et al. Catheter ablation in patients with multiple and unstable ventricular tachycardias after myocardial infarction: short ablation lines guided by reentry circuit isthmuses and sinus rhythm mapping. Circulation 2001;104:664–9.

5. Stevenson WG, Friedman PL, Kocovic D, et al. Radiofrequency catheter ablation of ventricular tachycardia after myocardial infarction. Circulation 1998;98:308–14.

6. Oza S, Wilber DJ. Substrate-based endocardial ablation of postinfarction ventricular tachycardia. Heart Rhythm 2006;3:607–9.

7. Verma A, Marrouche NF, Schweikert RA, et al. Relationship between successful ablation sites and the scar border zone defined by substrate mapping for ventricular tachycardia post-myocardial infarction. J Cardiovasc Electrophysiol 2005;16:465–71.

8. Brunken R, Tillisch J, Schwaiger M, et al. Regional perfusion, glucose metabolism, and wall motion in patients with chronic electrocardiographic Q wave infarctions: evidence for persistence of viable tissue in some infarct regions by positron emission tomography. Circulation 1986;73:951–63.

9. Maes A, Flameng W, Nuyts J, et al. Histological alterations in chronically hypoperfused myocardium. Correlation with PET findings. Circulation 1994;90:735–45.

10. Yoshida K, Gould KL. Quantitative relation of myocardial infarct size and myocardial viability by positron emission tomography to left ventricular ejection fraction and 3-year mortality with and without revascularization. J Am Coll Cardiol 1993; 22:984–97.

11. Tamaki N, Kawamoto M, Tadamura E, et al. Prediction of reversible ischemia after revascularization. Perfusion and metabolic studies with positron emission tomography. Circulation 1995;91:1697–705.

12. Dickfeld T, Calkins H, Zviman M, et al. Anatomic stereotactic catheter ablation on three-dimensional magnetic resonance images in real time. Circulation 2003;108:2407–13.

13. Fahmy TS, Wazni OM, Jaber WA, et al. Integration of positron emission tomography/computed tomography with electroanatomical mapping: a novel approach for ablation of scar-related ventricular tachycardia. Heart Rhythm 2008;5:1538–45.

14. Tian J, Smith MF, Chinnadurai P, et al. Clinical application of PET/CT fusion imaging for three-dimensional myocardial scar and left ventricular anatomy during ventricular tachycardia ablation. J Cardiovasc Electrophysiol 2008;20:597–604.

15. Tian J, Smith MF, Jeudy J, et al. Multimodality fusion imaging using delayed-enhanced cardiac magnetic resonance imaging, computed tomography, positron emission tomography and real-time intracardiac echocardiography to guide ventricular tachycardia ablation in implantable cardioverter-defibrillator patients. Heart Rhythm 2009;6:825–8.

16. Codreanu A, Odille F, Aliot E, et al. Electroanatomic characterization of post-infarct scars comparison with 3-dimensional myocardial scar reconstruction based on magnetic resonance imaging. J Am Coll Cardiol 2008;52:839–42.

17. Bogun FM, Desjardins B, Good E, et al. Delayed-enhanced magnetic resonance imaging in nonischemic cardiomyopathy: utility for identifying the ventricular arrhythmia substrate. J Am Coll Cardiol 2009;53:1138–45.

18. Desjardins B, Crawford T, Good E, et al. Infarct architecture and characteristics on delayed enhanced magnetic resonance imaging and electroanatomic mapping in patients with postinfarction ventricular arrhythmia. Heart Rhythm 2009;6:644–51.

19. de Bakker JM, van Capelle FJ, Janse MJ, et al. Reentry as a cause of ventricular tachycardia in patients with chronic ischemic heart disease: electrophysiologic and anatomic correlation. Circulation 1988;77:589–606.

20. de Bakker JM, van Capelle FJ, Janse MJ, et al. Slow conduction in the infarcted human heart. 'Zigzag' course of activation. Circulation 1993;88:915–26.

21. Tierney SP, Wilber DJ. Catheter ablation of ventricular tachycardia. Curr Treat Options Cardiovasc Med 2003;5:377–85.

22. Gepstein L, Hayam G, Ben-Haim SA. A novel method for nonfluoroscopic catheter-based electroanatomical mapping of the heart. In vitro and in vivo accuracy results. Circulation 1997;95:1611–22.

23. Stevenson WG, Wilber DJ, Natale A, et al. Irrigated radiofrequency catheter ablation guided by electroanatomic mapping for recurrent ventricular tachycardia after myocardial infarction: the Multicenter Thermocool Ventricular Tachycardia Ablation trial. Circulation 2000;118:2773–82.

24. Beanlands RS, Ruddy TD, deKemp RA, et al. Positron emission tomography and recovery following revascularization (PARR-1): the importance of scar and the development of a prediction rule for the degree of recovery of left ventricular function. J Am Coll Cardiol 2002;40:1735–43.

25. Maddahi J, Schelbert H, Brunken R, et al. Role of thallium-201 and PET imaging in evaluation of myocardial viability and management of patients

with coronary artery disease and left ventricular dysfunction. J Nucl Med 1994;35:707–15.

26. Cerqueira MD, Weissman NJ, Dilsizian V, et al. Standardized myocardial segmentation and nomenclature for tomographic imaging of the heart: a statement for healthcare professionals from the Cardiac Imaging Committee of the Council on Clinical Cardiology of the American Heart Association. J Nucl Cardiol 2002;9:240–5.

27. Tian J, Smith MF, Turgeman A, et al. Comparison of PET metabolic activities among scar, border zone and healthy myocardium in patients undergoing ischemic VT ablation. Heart Rhythm 2009;6:S165.

28. Tian J, Smith MF, Turgeman A, et al. Utilization of positron emission tomography perfusion/metabolic activities to predict electrophysiological voltage myocardium scar in patients undergoing ischemic ventricular tachycardia ablation. Circulation 2009;120:S388.

29. Dickfeld T, Lei P, Dilsizian V, et al. Integration of three-dimensional scar maps for ventricular tachycardia ablation using positron emission tomography/computed tomography (PET/CT). JACC Imaging 2008;1:73–82.

30. Cury RC, Nieman K, Shapiro MD, et al. Comprehensive assessment of myocardial perfusion defects, regional wall motion, and left ventricular function by using 64-section multidetector CT. Radiology 2008;248:466–75.

31. Fischbach R, Juergens KU, Ozgun M, et al. Assessment of regional left ventricular function with multidetector-row computed tomography versus magnetic resonance imaging. Eur Radiol 2007;17:1009–17.

32. Wu YW, Tadamura E, Yamamuro M, et al. Estimation of global and regional cardiac function using 64-slice computed tomography: a comparison study with echocardiography, gated-SPECT and cardiovascular magnetic resonance. Int J Cardiol 2008;128:69–76.

33. Tian J, Jeudy J, Smith MF, et al. Three dimensional contrast enhanced multi-detector CT for anatomic, dynamic and perfusion characterization of abnormal myocardium to guide VT ablations. Circ Arrhythm Electrophysiol 2010;3:495–504.

34. Kim RJ, Fieno DS, Parrish TB, et al. Relationship of MRI delayed contrast enhancement to irreversible injury, infarct age, and contractile function. Circulation 1999;100:1992–2002.

35. Wu E, Judd RM, Vargas JD, et al. Visualization of presence, location, and transmural extent of healed Q-wave and non-Q-wave myocardial infarction. Lancet 2001;357:21–8.

36. Rehwald WG, Fieno DS, Chen EL, et al. Myocardial magnetic resonance imaging contrast agent concentrations after reversible and irreversible ischemic injury. Circulation 2002;105:224–9.

37. Dickfeld T, Tian J, Ahmad G, et al. MRI-guided ventricular tachycardia ablation: integration of late gadolinium-enhanced 3D scar in patients with implantable cardioverter-defibrillators. Circ Arrhythm Electrophysiol 2011;4:172–84.

38. Faris OP, Shein M. Food and Drug Administration perspective: magnetic resonance imaging of pacemaker and implantable cardioverter-defibrillator patients. Circulation 2006;114:1232–3.

39. Marckmann P, Skov L, Rossen K, et al. Nephrogenic systemic fibrosis: suspected causative role of gadodiamide used for contrast-enhanced magnetic resonance imaging. J Am Soc Nephrol 2006;17:2359–62.

Emerging Role of Fluorodeoxyglucose-PET in the Diagnosis of Cardiac Sarcoidosis

Gagandeep S. Gurm, MD[a], Alin Chirindel, MD[b], Wengen Chen, MD, PhD[b],*

KEYWORDS

- FDG-PET • Cardiac sarcoidosis • Cardiac imaging

In the last 2 decades there has been significant development in cardiology, leading to better understanding and management of various disorders affecting the cardiovascular system. However, diagnosis of cardiac sarcoidosis (CS) still remains challenging. Noncaseating sarcoid granulomas can involve any region of the heart, namely the pericardium, myocardium, or endocardium, with the myocardium being the most frequently involved. Although the clinical literature suggests that less than 5% of patients with sarcoidosis may manifest clinical signs of cardiac involvement, autopsy studies have shown that subclinical cardiac involvement may be present in 20% to 25% of the patients.[1–4]

Some studies have reported that CS may be responsible for 13% to 25% deaths in patients with systemic sarcoidosis.[2] In the United States the lifetime risk of sarcoidosis is estimated to be 2.4% in blacks and 0.85% in whites.[5] This risk is higher outside the United States, with high incidence in Scandinavia, Ireland, and Japan. Cardiac involvement is more common in the Japanese population, especially in older women. Some studies have reported that more than 50% of deaths in sarcoidosis may be related to cardiac involvement.[5,6] This article discusses the role of cardiac images in the diagnosis of CS, with an emphasis on the emerging role of cardiac fluorodeoxyglucose (FDG)-PET.

CLINICAL PRESENTATION OF CS

Clinical presentation of CS can vary from subtle electrocardiographic changes to a more drastic picture as sudden cardiac death. Location and extent of granulomatous involvement are directly related to clinical presentation. Patients can commonly present with conduction abnormalities caused by involvement of the atrioventricular node or bundle of His. These abnormalities can initially present as first-degree heart block and then progress to complete heart blocks leading to syncope.[7,8]

Involvement of the ventricle can lead to reentrant arrhythmias, sustained or nonsustained ventricular tachycardias, and premature beats. Sudden cardiac death caused by ventricular tachyarrhythmias has been linked to 25% to 65% of deaths caused by CS, making early diagnosis essential.[1,9,10]

Extensive granulomatous infiltration of the myocardium can lead to heart failure in CS. Papillary muscle involvement can lead to valvular regurgitation, and lung involvement can further lead to right heart failure.[4] Diagnosis can be challenging,

The authors have nothing to disclose.

a Cardiology Division, Department of Medicine, Massachusetts General Hospital and Harvard Medical School, 55 Fruit Street, Boston, MA 02114, USA
b Department of Diagnostic Radiology and Nuclear Medicine, University of Maryland School of Medicine, 22 South Greene Street, Baltimore, MD 21201, USA
* Corresponding author.
E-mail address: wchen5@umm.edu

PET Clin 6 (2011) 403–408
doi:10.1016/j.cpet.2011.08.001

especially in the absence of diagnosis of systemic sarcoidosis. Pericardial effusions, symptomatic pericarditis, and constrictive pericarditis have also been reported.[11] Because early corticosteroid therapy can improve outcomes in these patients, early and accurate diagnosis is crucial.

Diagnosis

Because of the relatively high incidence of CS in Japan, the Japanese Ministry of Health and Welfare (JMH) has put together guidelines to establish the diagnosis of CS.[12] These guidelines are the only published schema for the diagnosis of CS. The guidelines either use endomyocardial biopsy (EB) for the histologic diagnosis or various diagnostic tests (radionuclide scintigraphy, echocardiography, electrocardiography [ECG], cardiac catheterization) for clinical diagnosis. The imaging studies help to identify ventricular dysfunction or perfusion defects. However, all these abnormalities are present only in late stages of the disease, hence making recovery unlikely.

ECG is a widely available inexpensive test. ECG has a low sensitivity and specificity for diagnosis of CS.[13,14] However, an abnormal ECG test in a patient with known extra-CS should trigger further evaluation. Patients with CS have a high prevalence of conduction abnormalities, ranging more than 50% in some studies.[15,16] The conduction system can be affected at any level, leading to atrioventricular blocks and even complete heart block. Patients can present with various ventricular arrhythmias, including sudden cardiac death, which makes it important to diagnose CS early.

EB can be useful by confirming the presence of granulomas or scarring and especially for excluding other causes of cardiac disease. EB is an invasive procedure with risk of serious complications. Moreover, although it is highly specific for CS, its sensitivity is low because of the heterogeneous involvement of the myocardium.[4,17] As a result, many patients with a strong clinical suspicion for CS and a negative biopsy are still treated for CS. Cardiac imaging modalities can play a crucial role in helping to identify a myocardial region, which can yield more specific results on EB.

ROLE OF CARDIAC IMAGING
Echocardiography

Many studies have shown a high prevalence of echocardiographic abnormalities in patients with sarcoidosis.[18–20] These abnormalities may include regional wall motion abnormalities, pericardial effusion, valvular regurgitations, and left ventricular systolic and diastolic dysfunction. However, these findings are nonspecific for CS, and further examinations are always needed to rule out other possibilities such as coronary artery disease. The echocardiographic abnormalities are likely present in later stages of the disease with myocardial scar formation. Utilization of echocardiography is thus limited in detecting early myocardial involvement.

Radionuclide techniques

Technetium 99m (^{99m}Tc)–labeled cardiac perfusion tracers and thallium 201 (^{201}Tl) have been used to detect cardiac involvement in sarcoidosis and are included in the JMH guidelines.[12] Sarcoidosis can lead to fibrogranulomatous replacement of the myocardium, leading to decreased uptake of the radiotracer in those regions.[21,22] Rarely the perfusion defect noted on rest images may show improvement on stress images, leading to so-called reverse distribution.[22,23] In a small study including 13 patients, a strong correlation was found in the extent of reverse redistribution and degree of improvement on follow-up studies after corticoid treatment.[22] Reverse redistribution is a rare phenomenon. The perfusion images are more commonly used to detect resting perfusion abnormalities. Other causes of perfusion defects such as coronary artery disease have to be excluded with the help of coronary angiography. As is the case with echocardiography these defects may represent late stages of CS with scar tissue formation and thus no improvement on treatment. With the JMH guidelines as the gold standard, the sensitivity of ^{201}Tl or ^{99m}Tc for detection of CS ranges from 50% to 60%.[22]

Gallium 67 (^{67}Ga) can accumulate in regions of active inflammation. ^{67}Ga can be taken up by inflammation caused by fibrogranulomatous involvement of the myocardium in CS. The reported sensitivity of ^{67}Ga scintigraphy ranges from 18% to 50% compared with myocardial perfusion imaging techniques.[4,24] Small studies have also shown improvement in uptake of ^{67}Ga after treatment with corticosteroids, thus suggesting its usefulness as a follow-up technique.[4]

Magnetic Resonance Imaging

Fibrogranulomatous replacement of the myocardium in CS can lead to delayed gadolinium (Gd) enhancement on cardiac magnetic resonance (MR) images. Compared with the subendocardial involvement seen in ischemic heart disease, the pattern of late Gd enhancement in CS involves midmyocardial regions. The high-resolution MR images can also be used to evaluate wall motion abnormalities and areas of focal thickening or thinning.[25–27] However, as the late Gd enhancement correlates with absence of viable myocytes, this technique detects only late stages of CS with limited recovery. Edema associated with inflammation is seen as increased signal intensity on both T2-weighted and early Gd enhancement images, representing early sarcoid involvement.[26] In studies involving small patient numbers the sensitivity and specificity of cardiac MR to detect sarcoid involvement range from 75% to 100% and 75% to 80%, respectively.[4,27] Similar to other imaging modalities cardiac MR findings also show improvement after treatment with corticosteroids.

EMERGING ROLE OF [^{18}F]FDG-PET

Metabolic PET imaging with the glucose analogue [^{18}F]FDG has been widely used in oncology and cardiac viability assessment. FDG accumulates in regions of increased glycolysis, distinguishing malignant tissue from normal surroundings. It also accumulates in regions with active inflammation such as lungs and hilar lymph nodes in patients with sarcoidosis.[28,29] These findings led investigators to evaluate the role of FDG-PET in the detection of CS involvement. **Table 1** lists the roles of FDG-PET, Cardiac MR, SPECT perfusion and Gallium scan in diagnosis of different stages of CS.

In addition to metabolic images, PET provides additional advantages of being able to acquire perfusion information. Thus, FDG uptake can provide a measurement of disease activity with perfusion images providing information about the extent of fibrogranulomatous replacement of the myocardium. In the first such study, Yamagishi and colleagues[30] studied the role of FDG-PET in 17 patients with biopsy proven systemic sarcoidosis. Out of the 17, 14 patients were noted to have increased FDG uptake on PET. Of these patients, 7 underwent repeat FDG-PET 1 month after treatment with steroids. These investigators found marked decrease in the extent and intensity of FDG uptake in 5 patients and complete resolution of FDG uptake in 2 patients.

Okumura and colleagues[31] compared FDG-PET with the JMH guidelines for detection of CS. They divided 22 patients with systemic sarcoidosis into 2 groups of 11 patients each according to the presence or absence of CS in accordance with the JMH guidelines. Standardized uptake value (SUV) of FDG-PET was used to quantify myocardial uptake. All the patients also underwent ^{99m}Tc-hexakis-2-methoxyisobutylisonitrile (MIBI) myocardium single-photon emission computed tomography (SPECT) and ^{67}Ga scintigraphy imaging. When all the imaging modalities were compared with JMH guidelines for the detection of CS, FDG-PET had a sensitivity of 100%, whereas the sensitivity for ^{99m}Tc-MIBI SPECT and ^{67}Ga scintigraphy was

63.6% and 36.3%, respectively. Also in patients with CS FDG-PET images showed a higher prevalence of abnormal uptake than defects detected on ^{99m}Tc-MIBI SPECT images ($P<.05$), suggesting that FDG-PET can detect early myocardial involvement.

Although these initial small studies suggest that FDG-PET cardiac imaging may be a promising technique for the diagnosis and management of CS, there are still many unanswered questions. One of these crucial questions is whether the focal uptake of FDG is pathologic or just a normal variant. Studies have previously reported that focal abnormal FDG uptake in the myocardium is nonspecific and can be seen in a significant number of patients with idiopathic dilated cardiomyopathy.[32,33] This question was addressed by Ishimura and colleagues.[34] These investigators took 32 patients with sarcoidosis and compared their FDG-PET uptake with 30 control subjects. They found that the control subjects either had no FDG uptake (n = 16) or had diffuse FDG uptake (n = 14). In contrast, 15 subjects with sarcoidosis showed none, 7 showed diffuse, 8 showed focal, and 2 showed focal on diffuse patterns, with the prevalence of the focal and focal on diffuse patterns being significantly higher in the sarcoidosis group when compared with the control group ($P<.001$). Thus these investigators concluded that focal uptake of the heart on [^{18}F]FDG-PET images is a characteristic feature of patients with sarcoidosis.

The myocardium has a unique ability to switch substrate according to the metabolic needs. Under normal resting conditions, 65% to 70% of the energy is provided by long chain fatty acids and 15% to 20% is generally provided by glucose. The myocardium may have varying degrees of FDG uptake under resting conditions, which can highly reduce the specificity for CS imaging. To have the best accuracy, one of the challenges is to minimize the normal FDG uptake in the myocardium. Various techniques have been suggested, including a diet rich in fatty acids and low in carbohydrates at least for the 24 hours before the imaging. This method has been suggested to decrease FDG uptake in the myocardium.[35] Some researchers have suggested the use of unfractionated heparin infusion before FDG injection. Unfractionated heparin has been shown to enhance the plasma lipolytic activity, increasing the plasma free fatty acid levels and forcing myocardium to use free fatty acids.[36] Another study has suggested that prolonged fasting for more than 18 hours can also decrease the amount of normal FDG uptake in the myocardium.[37] None of these techniques has been studied widely and more studies are needed for their validation.

Table 1
Possible role of various cardiac imaging modalities in diagnosis of different stages of CS

Modality	Early	Intermediate	Late
PET	Focal increased FDG uptake	Focal/heterogeneous uptake of FDG	No FDG uptake, suggesting scar
Cardiac MR	Myocardial edema	Edema/delayed enhancement	Delayed enhancement suggesting scar
SPECT perfusion	Reverse Redistribution (rare)	Decreased radiotracer uptake	No radiotracer uptake in scarred myocardium
Ga	Increased uptake	May show increased uptake	No uptake

FDG-PET can also be used to follow treatment response in patients with CS. In the study by Yamagishi and colleagues,[30] 7 patients underwent repeat FDG-PET 1 month after treatment with steroids. These investigators found a marked decrease in the extent and intensity of FDG uptake in 5 patients and complete resolution of FDG uptake in 2 patients. **Fig. 1** shows FDG-PET images from a patient at our institution before and after treatment with steroids.

Compared with other imaging modalities FDG-PET has shown a higher sensitivity for the detection of CS.[31,37] Only 1 study has compared FDG-PET with cardiac MR for this purpose. In this study by Ohira and colleagues,[36] patients with suspected CS underwent FDG-PET and

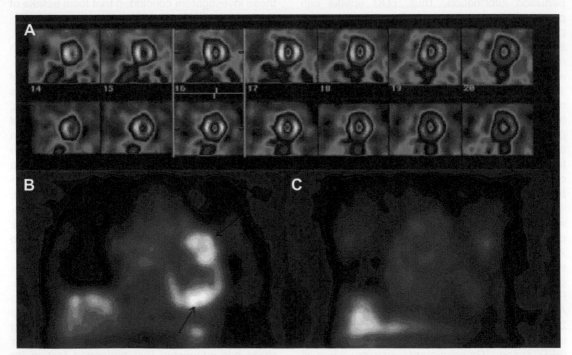

Fig. 1. Images from a 42-year-old woman with biopsy proven neurosarcoidosis who presented with ventricular tachycardia. (*A*) Myocardial perfusion single-photon emission tomography images; stress (*top row*) and rest (*bottom row*) showed normal perfusion. (*B*) FDG-PET image showed focal uptake in the midanterior and midinferior region of the myocardium, suggesting sarcoidosis involvement. (*C*) Follow-up FDG-PET images showed resolution of focal FDG uptake after steroid treatment.

cardiac MR imaging. Taking JMH guidelines as the gold standard for diagnosis of CS, the sensitivity and specificity for diagnosis of CS was 87.5% and 38.5%, respectively, for FDG-PET and 75% and 76.9%, respectively, for cardiac MR imaging.[36]

SUMMARY

Despite significant development in cardiac imaging, diagnosis of CS remains challenging. Autopsy studies have shown that up to 25% of patients with systemic sarcoidosis may have cardiac involvement predisposing them to fatal arrhythmias. Thus accurate and early diagnosis of CS is highly relevant. Radionuclide techniques using ^{99m}Tc, ^{201}Tl, and ^{67}Ga are among the oldest imaging methods used to diagnose CS. Other techniques such as MR imaging and echocardiography have also been used to help evaluate CS involvement. More recently, metabolic PET with glucose analogue [^{18}F]FDG has been used to image CS. FDG accumulates in the regions of inflammation with increased glycolysis, making it an ideal tracer for imaging CS and treatment follow-up. However, the data are limited and most of these studies are small and retrospective in nature. Large prospective studies are needed in future to further establish the role of FDG-PET in this arena. FDG-PET imaging may evolve as a promising technique for accurate and early diagnosis of CS.

REFERENCES

1. Robert WC, McAllister HA Jr, Ferrans VJ. Sarcoidosis of the heart, A clinicopathologic study of 35 necropsy patients (group 1) and review of 78 previously described necropsy patients (group 2). Am J Med 1977;63:86–108.
2. Silverman KJ, Hutchins GM, Bulkley BH. Cardiac sarcoid: a clinicopathologic study of 84 unselected patients with systemic sarcoidosis. Circulation 1978;58:1204–11.
3. Tavora F, Cresswell N, Li L, et al. Comparison of necropsy findings in patients with sarcoidosis dying suddenly from cardiac sarcoidosis versus dying suddenly from other causes. Am J Cardiol 2009; 104:571–7.
4. Kim JS, Judson MA, Donnino R, et al. Cardiac sarcoidosis. Am Heart J 2009;157:9–21.
5. Rybicki BA, Major M, Popovich J Jr, et al. Racial differences in sarcoidosis incidence: a 5-year study in a health maintenance organization. Am J Epidemiol 1997;145:234–41.
6. Iwai K, Sekiguti M, Hosoda Y, et al. Racial difference in cardiac sarcoidosis incidence observed at autopsy. Sarcoidosis 1994;11:26–31.
7. Chapelon-Abric C, de Zuttere D, Duhaut P, et al. Cardiac sarcoidosis: a retrospective study of 41 cases. Medicine (Baltimore) 2004;83:315–34.
8. Yoshida Y, Morimoto S, Hiramitsu S, et al. Incidence of cardiac sarcoidosis in Japanese patients with high-degree atrioventricular block. Am Heart J 1997;134:382–6.
9. Yazaki Y, Isobe M, Hiroe M, et al. Prognostic determinants of long-term survival in Japanese patients with cardiac sarcoidosis treated with prednisone. Am J Cardiol 2001;88:1006–10.
10. Reuhl J, Schneider M, Sievert H, et al. Myocardial sarcoidosis as a rare cause of sudden cardiac death. Forensic Sci Int 1997;89:145–53.
11. Garrett J, O'Neill H, Blake S. Constrictive pericarditis associated with sarcoidosis. Am Heart J 1984; 107:394.
12. Hiraga H, Yuwa K, Hiroe M. Guidelines for the diagnosis of cardiac sarcoidosis: study report on diffuse pulmonary disease. Jpn Ministry Health Welfare 1993;88:23–4.
13. Sekiguchi M, Yazaki Y, Isobe M, et al. Cardiac sarcoidosis: diagnostic, prognostic, and therapeutic considerations. Cardiovasc Drugs Ther 1996;10: 495–510.
14. Numao Y, Sekiguchi M, Hirosawa K, et al. Evaluation of cardiac involvement through electrocardiogram in patients with sarcoidosis. Kokyu To Junkan 1981;29: 421–8.
15. Fleming HA, Bailey SM. Sarcoid heart disease. J R Coll Physicians Lond 1981;15:245–6, 249–53.
16. Matsui Y, Iwai K, Tachibana T, et al. Clinicopathological study of fatal myocardial sarcoidosis. Ann N Y Acad Sci 1976;278:455–69.
17. Uemura A, Morimoto S, Hiramitsu S, et al. Histologic diagnostic rate of cardiac sarcoidosis: evaluation of endomyocardial biopsies. Am Heart J 1999;138: 299–302.
18. Kinney EL, Jackson GL, Reeves WC, et al. Thallium-scan myocardial defects and echocardiographic abnormalities in patients with sarcoidosis without clinical cardiac dysfunction. Am J Med 1980;68: 497–503.
19. Lewin RF, Mor R, Spitzer S, et al. Echocardiographic evaluation of patients with systemic sarcoidosis. Am Heart J 1985;110:116–22.
20. Burstow DJ, Tajik J, Baily KR, et al. Two-dimensional echocardiographic findings in systemic sarcoidosis. Am J Cardiol 1989;63:497–503.
21. Bulkley BH, Rouleau JB, Whitaker JQ, et al. The use of 201thallium for myocardial perfusion imaging in sarcoid heart disease. Chest 1977;72:27–32.
22. Le Guludec D, Menad F, Faraggi M, et al. Myocardial sarcoidosis. Clinical value of technetium-99m

sestamibi tomoscintigraphy. Chest 1994;106: 1675–82.

23. Haywood LJ, Sharma OP, Siegel ME, et al. Detection of myocardial sarcoidosis by thallium 201 imaging. J Natl Med Assoc 1982;74:959–64.

24. Fields G, Ossorio M, Roy T, et al. Thallium 201 scintigraphy in the diagnosis and management of myocardial sarcoidosis. South Med J 1990;83:339–42.

25. Vignaux O, Dhote R, Dudoc D, et al. Detection of myocardial involvement in patients with sarcoidosis applying T2-weighted, contrast-enhanced, and cine magnetic resonance imaging: initial results of a prospective study. J Comput Assist Tomogr 2002;26:762–7.

26. Vignaux O. Cardiac sarcoidosis: spectrum of MRI features. AJR Am J Roentgenol 2005;184:249–54.

27. Smedema JP, Snoep G, Van Kroonenburgh MP, et al. Evaluation of the accuracy of gadolinium-enhanced cardiovascular magnetic resonance in the diagnosis of cardiac sarcoidosis. J Am Coll Cardiol 2005;45:1683–90.

28. Brudin LH, Valind S, Rhodes CG, et al. Fluorine-18 deoxyglucose uptake in sarcoidosis measured with positron emission tomography. Eur J Nucl Med 1994;21:297–305.

29. Lewis P, Salama A. Uptake of fluorine-18-fluorodeoxyglucose in sarcoidosis. J Nucl Med 1994;35:1647–9.

30. Yamagishi H, Shirai N, Takagi M, et al. Identification of cardiac sarcoidosis with 13N-NH3/18F-FDG PET. J Nucl Med 2003;44:1030–6.

31. Okumura W, Iwasaki T, Toyama T, et al. Usefulness of fasting 18F-FDG PET in identification of cardiac sarcoidosis. J Nucl Med 2004;45:1989–98.

32. Yokoyama I, Momomura S, Ohtake T, et al. Role of positron emission tomography using fluorine-18 fluoro-2-deoxyglucose in predicting improvement in left ventricular function in patients with idiopathic dilated cardiomyopathy. Eur J Nucl Med 1998;25:736–43.

33. Van den Heuvel AF, van Veldhuisen DJ, van der Wall EE, et al. Regional myocardial blood flow reserve impairment and metabolic changes suggesting myocardial ischemia in patients with idiopathic dilated cardiomyopathy. J Am Coll Cardiol 2000;35:19–28.

34. Ishimaru S, Tsujino I, Takei T, et al. Focal uptake of 18F-fluoro-2-deoxyglucose positron emission tomography images indicates cardiac involvement of sarcoidosis. Eur Heart J 2005;26:1538–43.

35. Williams G, Kolodny GM. Suppression of myocardial 18F-FDG uptake by preparing patients with a high fat, low carbohydrate diet. AJR Am J Roentgenol 2008;190:1406–9.

36. Ohira H, Tsujino I, Ishimaru S, et al. Myocardial imaging with 18F-fluoro-2-deoxyglucose positron emission tomography and magnetic resonance imaging in sarcoidosis. Eur J Nucl Med Mol Imaging 2008;35:933–41.

37. Langah R, Spicer K, Gebregziabher M, et al. Effectiveness of prolonged fasting 18F-FDG PET-CT in the detection of cardiac sarcoidosis. J Nucl Cardiol 2009;16:801–10.

Detection and Quantification of Molecular Calcification by PET/Computed Tomography: A New Paradigm in Assessing Atherosclerosis

Babak Saboury, MD, MPH, Pouya Ziai, MD,
Abass Alavi, MD, PhD (Hon), DSc (Hon)*

KEYWORDS

- Molecular calcification • ^{18}F-Sodium fluoride
- Atherogenesis • Atherosclerosis

Atherosclerosis is the leading cause of cardiovascular events. Formation of atherosclerotic plaque is a dynamic process that includes distinctive pathophysiologic stages. According to the American Heart Association (AHA), there are 6 stages of atherosclerotic plaque development in human (**Fig. 1**), with inflammation being prominent in the early stages and calcification in the later stages.[1] Atherosclerotic plaque disruption is considered to be the most frequent cause of sudden cardiovascular events. However, the exact characteristics of the plaque, which make it vulnerable to rupture and subsequent cardiovascular events, have not been fully understood, and it still remains an unknown phenomenon. Inflammation and microcalcification, as two distinctive features of atherogenesis, have been hypothesized to play potential roles in enhancing plaque vulnerability and subsequent rupture.[2–4] On the other hand calcification, when it becomes substantial, has also been suggested to result in plaque stability.[5,6]

It therefore seems clear that there is a dire need to develop innovative noninvasive imaging technologies to identify characteristics of the atherosclerotic plaque that may be able to reveal any relation among various stages of atherosclerosis and cardiovascular events and that would allow definition of the nature of vulnerable plaques. Plaque vulnerability has been shown to primarily reflect the cellular and extracellular composition rather than the size of the plaque or the degree of luminal narrowing.[7,8] So angiography, the current gold-standard imaging modality for imaging the vascular tree, which can only provide structural details in symptomatic arterial stenosis, is not useful in identifying nonstenotic, inflamed plaques that are prone to future rupture.[9] Therefore, an optimal preventive strategy in reducing cardiovascular morbidity and mortality would be not only to detect atherosclerotic lesions but also to identify asymptomatic patients who are prone to plaque rupture and who would benefit the most from intensive, evidence-based medical interventions.[10,11] Being able to identify

Department of Radiology, School of Medicine, University of Pennsylvania, 3400 Spruce Street, Philadelphia, PA 19104, USA
* Corresponding author.
E-mail address: Abass.Alavi@uphs.upenn.edu

PET Clin 6 (2011) 409–415
doi:10.1016/j.cpet.2011.10.001

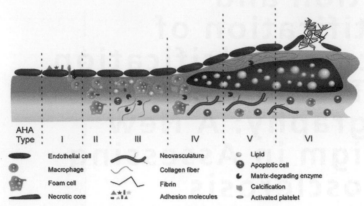

Fig. 1. The different stages of atherosclerotic plaque development in humans. AHA, American Heart Association. (*From* Douma K, Prinzen L, Slaaf DW, et al. Nanoparticles for optical molecular imaging of atherosclerosis. Small 2009;5(5):544–57; with permission.)

and quantify inflammation and molecular calcification, modern molecular imaging techniques and those related to PET have the ability to provide sufficient information about various stages of atheroma. In particular, ^{18}F-fluorodeoxyglucose (FDG) PET/computed tomography (CT) imaging is now considered a well-established and reliable method in detecting and quantifying the process of cellular inflammation.[12–17] Similarly, ^{18}F-sodium fluoride (^{18}F-NaF) recently has been shown to be the tracer of choice for the detection of molecular calcification in the heart and arterial wall.[18]

ROLE OF ^{18}F-FLUORIDE PET IN IMAGING OF ATHEROSCLEROSIS

[18]F-NaF is a position-emitting radiotracer that was introduced by Blau and colleagues[19] in 1962 to assess new bone formation in normal and pathologic states. The US Food and Drug Administration approved it for clinical use in 1972.[20] ^{18}F-NaF can be readily taken up from blood at sites of active calcification and new bone formation, and is rapidly cleared from blood in a biexponential manner, which results in a high bone-to-background ratio in a short time.[20] Retention of ^{18}F-NaF by the bone has 2 phases. First the [18]F$^-$ ion exchanges for the OH$^-$ ion on the surface of the bone, and next it incorporates into the crystalline matrix of the bone and is retained there until the bone is remodeled.[21] Because of these favorable pharmacokinetic characteristics, there is a large number of studies depicting the utility of ^{18}F-NaF–PET/CT in assessing malignant and benign disorders of the skeletal system.[22–25] Of interest, the process of calcification in atherosclerosis has been shown to have remarkable similarities to the formation of new bone and to

share the similar cell types, signaling pathways, and metabolic compounds.[26–28]

In the animal study performed by the authors' group, the utility of ^{18}F-NaF in detecting molecular calcification of heart and major vessels of diabetic pigs was evaluated. These animals were examined at different stages of the disease with both ^{18}F-FDG and ^{18}F-NaF. Using ^{18}F-NaF, the authors were able to visualize molecular calcification in the heart and lower lumbar aorta of diabetic pigs far in advance of visualization of any visible calcification in the CT images (**Fig. 2**), which indicates that ^{18}F-NaF PET can offer the advantage of providing highly relevant information about the characteristics of calcified plaque long before it will be detectable by CT (University of Pennsylvania, unpublished data).

Recently, the utility of FDG along with ^{18}F-NaF in functional imaging of arterial wall alterations was described by some researchers. In a retrospective study, Derlin and colleagues[29] evaluated 75 patients who had undergone whole-body ^{18}F-NaF–PET/CT for the exclusion of bone metastasis, to examine the prevalence, location, and topographic relationship of ^{18}F-NaF accumulation and vascular calcification in major arteries. Using visual and semiquantitative analysis they were able to show that 88% of the lesions with ^{18}F-NaF uptake had concordant evidence for calcification in the thoracic aorta and at the carotid bifurcation by CT (**Fig. 3**). In addition, this study showed that a higher degree of calcification is related to the higher probability of ^{18}F-NaF uptake visibility; however the investigators found no significant correlation between the intensity of radiotracer uptake (maximum standardized uptake value or SUV$_{max}$) and the calcification score. This study also showed that colocalization of ^{18}F-NaF uptake

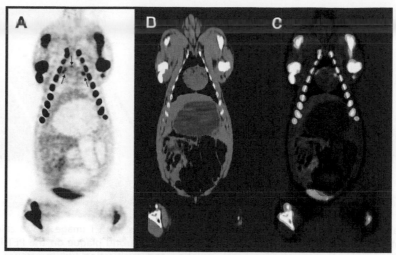

Fig. 2. Coronal ^{18}F-NaF–PET/CT images of a diabetic pig with known atherosclerotic lesions. (A) PET image generated 1 hour after the administration of ^{18}F-NaF. Black arrows represent 3 sites of calcification either in the coronary arteries or in the soft tissues of the myocardium. (B) There is no or minimal evidence of calcification at these sites on the CT image. (C) Fused PET/CT image shows the location of cardiac calcification.

and CT calcification is substantially higher than previously reported colocalization of ^{18}F-FDG and CT calcification.[14,30,31] Another study by Derlin and colleagues[32] evaluated the correlation between ^{18}F-NaF and arterial wall calcification in the common carotid arteries. In this study, they semiquantitatively measured the SUV$_{max}$ by placing an individual region of interest (ROI) around the lesion on coregistered transaxial PET/CT images. Using this method they showed a significant correlation between ^{18}F-NaF uptake and arterial wall calcification, and also between degree of radiotracer uptake (SUV$_{max}$) and both calcification score and calcified lesion thickness in the atherosclerotic plaque (**Fig. 4**). These investigators also showed that ^{18}F-NaF uptake in calcifying carotid plaque has significant correlation

with cardiovascular risk factors such as age (P = .0001), gender (male sex, P = .0001), hypertension (P = .002), hypercholesterolemia (P = .05), and cumulative smoking exposure (P = .02). In addition, they showed that an increase in the number of these risk factors is associated with an increase in the percentage of patients with F-NaF accumulation.

In one more study by the same group of researchers, both ^{18}F-FDG and ^{18}F-NaF were used to evaluate different stages of atherosclerosis with regard to the age of the atherosclerotic lesion (**Fig. 5**). Semiquantitative analysis was performed by obtaining the SUV$_{max}$. The ROI was placed manually around the lesion on coregistered transaxial PET/CT images. Colocalization of ^{18}F-NaF uptake and CT calcification was 77.1%, which is

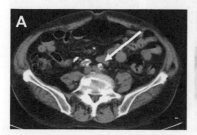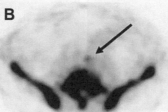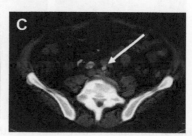

Fig. 3. Transaxial ^{18}F-NaF–PET/CT images of common iliac arteries. (A) CT image. White arrow shows calcification. (B) There is an ^{18}F-NaF uptake indicated by a black arrow on the PET image. (C) Fused PET/CT image shows colocalization of ^{18}F-NaF uptake and calcification in atherosclerotic lesion (*white arrow*). (*From* Derlin T, Richter U, Bannas P, et al. Feasibility of 18F-sodium fluoride PET/CT for imaging of atherosclerotic plaque. J Nucl Med 2010;51(6):862–5; with permission.)

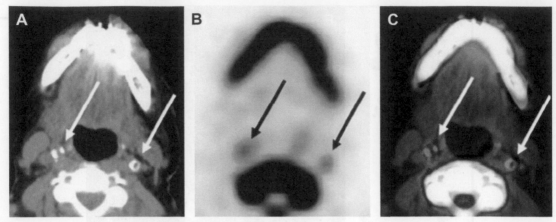

Fig. 4. Transaxial ^{18}F-NaF–PET/CT images of common carotid arteries. (*A*) CT image shows calcification (*white arrows*). (*B*) Bilateral ^{18}F-NaF uptake indicated by black arrows in carotid plaque on the PET image. (*C*) Fused PET/CT image shows colocalization of ^{18}F-naF accumulation and calcification (*white arrows*). (*From* Derlin T, Wisotzki C, Richter U, et al. In vivo imaging of mineral deposition in carotid plaque using 18F-sodium fluoride PET/CT: correlation with atherogenic risk factors. J Nucl Med 2011;52(3):362–8; with permission.)

significantly higher than colocalization of FDG and CT calcification (14.5%). Also, ^{18}F-FDG and ^{18}F-NaF tracer accumulation was colocalized in only 6.5% of lesions, indicating that these tracers identify different and distinct features of atherogenesis.[33]

In a novel study performed by their group, the authors described for the first time the feasibility of ^{18}F-NaF–PET/CT for the quantification of global molecular calcification of the heart and aorta.[18] The authors examined the image data sets of 51 patients who had undergone ^{18}F-NaF–PET/CT for evaluation of a variety of malignancies. For quantitative analysis of PET images, an ellipsoid ROI was assigned to cardiac silhouette on each slice of CT and corresponding PET slice all over the heart (**Fig. 6**). Then the volume of each slice was calculated by multiplying the area on the ROI by the slice

thickness, and mean standardized uptake value (SUV$_{mean}$) of each ROI was generated. Finally, by adding the molecular calcification scores among the entire set of calculated ROI, the cardiac Global Molecular Calcification Score (GMCS) was generated. This method was inspired by the global disease assessment concept, first described in Alzheimer disease in 1993.[34] Subjects were categorized in 5 age groups (<40, 41–50, 51–60, 61–70, >70 years). The Pearson correlation coefficient for correlation between mean cardiac GMCS and mean of aortic SUV$_{mean}$ on one side and the 5 age groups on the other side was 0.92 (*P* = .003) and 0.97 (*P* = .004), respectively (**Figs. 7** and **8**).

Using this method, the authors showed that global measurement of ^{18}F-NaF uptake in the heart and aorta could be used to detect and quantify molecular calcification in these structures. The

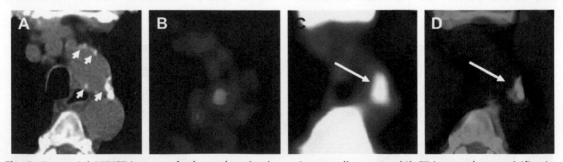

Fig. 5. Transaxial PET/CT images of atherosclerotic plaque in ascending aorta: (*A*) CT image shows calcification (*short arrows*). (*B*) ^{18}F-FDG PET image shows no tracer uptake; however, on ^{18}F-NaF PET image (*C*) there is an accumulation of tracer indicated by a long arrow. (*D*) Coregistered and fused ^{18}F-FDG/^{18}F-NaF PET/CT (*long arrow*). (*From* Derlin T, Toth Z, Papp L, et al. Correlation of inflammation assessed by 18F-FDG PET, active mineral deposition assessed by 18F-fluoride PET, and vascular calcification in atherosclerotic plaque: a dual-tracer PET/CT study. J Nucl Med 2011;52(7):1020–7; with permission.)

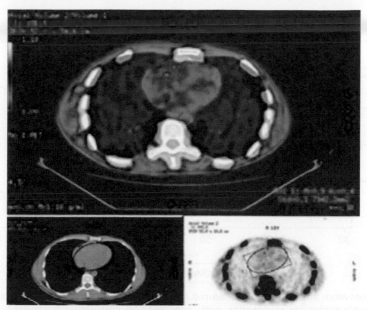

Fig. 6. Atypical region of interest (ROI) that was drawn around the ventricles on each slice of CT and the corresponding PET slice. Here the volume of the selected ROI volume was 30.8 cm^3 in this particular slice, and the mean standardized uptake value (SUV$_{mean}$) on the corresponding PET slice was 0.5. Therefore, the molecular calcification score was calculated to be 15.4 (30.8 × 0.5 = 15.4) for this particular slice. Using this approach the Global Calcification Score for the entire heart was calculated. (*From* Beheshti M, Saboury B, Mehta N, et al. Detection and global quantification of cardiovascular molecular calcification by fluoro-18-fluoride positron emission tomography/computed tomography—A novel concept. Hell J Nucl Med 2011;14(2);114–20; with permission.)

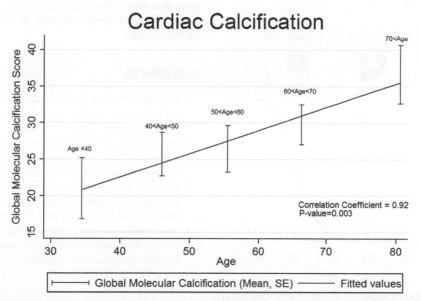

Fig. 7. Correlation between cardiac Global Molecular Calcification Score (GMCS), measured by^{18}F-NaF–PET/CT, and age. There is a statistically significant increase in cardiac molecular calcification with age (Pearson correlation coefficient = 0.92; P = .003). (*From* Beheshti M, Saboury B, Mehta N, et al. Detection and global quantification of cardiovascular molecular calcification by fluoro-18-fluoride positron emission tomography/computed tomography—A novel concept. Hell J Nucl Med 2011;14(2);114–20; with permission.)

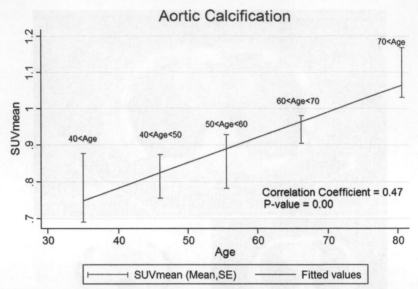

Fig. 8. Correlation between aortic SUV$_{mean}$, measured by[18]F-NaF-PET/CT, and age. There is a statistically significant increase in aortic molecular calcification with age (Pearson correlation coefficient = 0.97; P = .004). (*From* Beheshti M, Saboury B, Mehta N, et al. Detection and global quantification of cardiovascular molecular calcification by fluoro-18-fluoride positron emission tomography/computed tomography—A novel concept. Hell J Nucl Med 2011;14(2);114–20; with permission.)

study showed that ^{18}F-NaF–PET/CT is able to identify and evaluate the properties of atherosclerotic plaque early on in its course in the heart and aorta; and age, as the most potent risk factor of atherosclerosis, was shown to have significant correlation with the level of molecular calcification in these structures.[18]

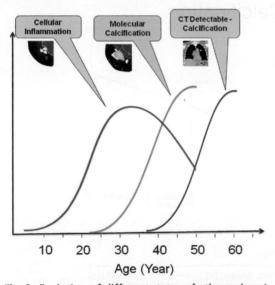

Fig. 9. Evolution of different states of atherosclerosis over time. Inflammation is followed by molecular calcification and CT calcification years later. Molecular imaging with PET is able to detect and quantify the cellular inflammation and molecular calcification long before irreversible CT calcification is made.

SUMMARY

Detection and quantification of molecular calcification by NaF can bridge the gap between cellular inflammation detected by FDG and visible calcification identified by CT (**Fig. 9**). However, further prospective studies are needed to evaluate the potential role of this approach in elucidating pathophysiology of atherosclerosis at different stages of the disease.

REFERENCES

1. Douma K, Prinzen L, Slaaf DW, et al. Nanoparticles for optical molecular imaging of atherosclerosis. Small 2009;5(5):544–57.
2. Bluestein D, Alemu Y, Avrahami I, et al. Influence of microcalcifications on vulnerable plaque mechanics using FSI modeling. J Biomech 2008;41(5):1111–8.
3. Libby P, Ridker PM, Hansson GK. Progress and challenges in translating the biology of atherosclerosis. Nature 2011;473(7347):317–25.
4. Vengrenyuk Y, Carlier S, Xanthos S, et al. A hypothesis for vulnerable plaque rupture due to stress-induced debonding around cellular microcalcifications in thin fibrous caps. Proc Natl Acad Sci U S A 2006;103(40):14678–83.
5. Huang H, Virmani R, Younis H, et al. The impact of calcification on the biomechanical stability of atherosclerotic plaques. Circulation 2001;103(8):1051–6.
6. Imoto K, Hiro T, Fujii T, et al. Longitudinal structural determinants of atherosclerotic plaque vulnerability: a computational analysis of stress distribution using vessel

models and three-dimensional intravascular ultrasound imaging. J Am Coll Cardiol 2005;46(8):1507–15.

7. Ambrose JA, Tannenbaum MA, Alexopoulos D, et al. Angiographic progression of coronary artery disease and the development of myocardial infarction. J Am Coll Cardiol 1988;12(1):56–62.

8. Little WC, Constantinescu M, Applegate RJ, et al. Can coronary angiography predict the site of a subsequent myocardial infarction in patients with mild-to-moderate coronary artery disease? Circulation 1988;78(5 Pt 1):1157–66.

9. Pasterkamp G, Schoneveld AH, van der Wal AC, et al. Relation of arterial geometry to luminal narrowing and histologic markers for plaque vulnerability: the remodeling paradox. J Am Coll Cardiol 1998;32(3):655–62.

10. Greenland P, Abrams J, Aurigemma GP, et al. Prevention Conference V: Beyond secondary prevention: identifying the high-risk patient for primary prevention: noninvasive tests of atherosclerotic burden: Writing Group III. Circulation 2000;101(1):E16–22.

11. Taylor AJ, Merz CN, Udelson JE. 34th Bethesda Conference: Executive summary—can atherosclerosis imaging techniques improve the detection of patients at risk for ischemic heart disease? J Am Coll Cardiol 2003;41(11):1860–2.

12. Rudd JH, Myers KS, Bansilal S, et al. Atherosclerosis inflammation imaging with ^{18}F-FDG PET: carotid, iliac, and femoral uptake reproducibility, quantification methods, and recommendations. J Nucl Med 2008;49(6):871–8.

13. Bural GG, Torigian DA, Chamroonrat W, et al. Quantitative assessment of the atherosclerotic burden of the aorta by combined FDG-PET and CT image analysis: a new concept. Nucl Med Biol 2006;33(8):1037–43.

14. Ben-Haim S, Kupzov V, Tamir A, et al. Evaluation of ^{18}F-FDG uptake and arterial wall calcifications using ^{18}F-FDG PET/CT. J Nucl Med 2004;45(11):1816–21.

15. Tatsumi M, Cohade C, Nakamoto Y, et al. Fluorodeoxyglucose uptake in the aortic wall at PET/CT: possible finding for active atherosclerosis. Radiology 2003;229(3):831–7.

16. Yun M, Jang S, Cucchiara A, et al. [18]F FDG uptake in the large arteries: a correlation study with the atherogenic risk factors. Semin Nucl Med 2002;32(1):70–6.

17. Yun M, Yeh D, Araujo LI, et al. F-18 FDG uptake in the large arteries: a new observation. Clin Nucl Med 2001;26(4):314–9.

18. Beheshti M, Saboury B, Mehta NN, et al. Detection and global quantification of cardiovascular molecular calcification by fluoro-18-fluoride positron emission tomography/computed tomography-A novel concept. Hell J Nucl Med 2011;14(2):114–20.

19. Blau M, Nagler W, Bender MA. Fluorine-18: a new isotope for bone scanning. J Nucl Med 1962;3:332–4.

20. Grant FD, Fahey F, Packard A, et al. Skeletal PET with ^{18}F-fluoride: applying new technology to an old tracer. J Nucl Med 2008;49(1):68–78.

21. Costeas A, Woodard HQ, Laughlin JS. Depletion of ^{18}F from blood flowing through bone. J Nucl Med 1970;11(1):43–5.

22. Lim R, Fahey FH, Drubach LA, et al. Early experience with fluorine-18 sodium fluoride bone PET in young patients with back pain. J Pediatr Orthop 2007;27(3):277–82.

23. Ovadia D, Metser U, Lievshitz G, et al. Back pain in adolescents: assessment with integrated ^{18}F-fluoride positron-emission tomography-computed tomography. J Pediatr Orthop 2007;27(1):90–3.

24. Schirrmeister H, Guhlmann A, Kotzerke J, et al. Early detection and accurate description of extent of metastatic bone disease in breast cancer with fluoride ion and positron emission tomography. J Clin Oncol 1999;17(8):2381–9.

25. Tse N, Hoh C, Hawkins R, et al. Positron emission tomography diagnosis of pulmonary metastases in osteogenic sarcoma. Am J Clin Oncol 1994;17(1):22–5.

26. Dhore CR, Cleutjens JP, Lutgens E, et al. Differential expression of bone matrix regulatory proteins in human atherosclerotic plaques. Arterioscler Thromb Vasc Biol 2001;21(12):1998–2003.

27. Doherty TM, Asotra K, Fitzpatrick LA, et al. Calcification in atherosclerosis: bone biology and chronic inflammation at the arterial crossroads. Proc Natl Acad Sci U S A 2003;100(20):11201–6.

28. Engelse MA, Neele JM, Bronckers AL, et al. Vascular calcification: expression patterns of the osteoblast-specific gene core binding factor alpha-1 and the protective factor matrix Gla protein in human atherogenesis. Cardiovasc Res 2001;52(2):281–9.

29. Derlin T, Richter U, Bannas P, et al. Feasibility of ^{18}F-sodium fluoride PET/CT for imaging of atherosclerotic plaque. J Nucl Med 2010;51(6):862–5.

30. Dunphy MP, Freiman A, Larson SM, et al. Association of vascular ^{18}F-FDG uptake with vascular calcification. J Nucl Med 2005;46(8):1278–84.

31. Ogawa M, Ishino S, Mukai T, et al. (18)F-FDG accumulation in atherosclerotic plaques: immunohistochemical and PET imaging study. J Nucl Med 2004;45(7):1245–50.

32. Derlin T, Wisotzki C, Richter U, et al. In vivo imaging of mineral deposition in carotid plaque using ^{18}F-sodium fluoride PET/CT: correlation with atherogenic risk factors. J Nucl Med 2011;52(3):362–8.

33. Derlin T, Toth Z, Papp L, et al. Correlation of inflammation assessed by ^{18}F-FDG PET, active mineral deposition assessed by ^{18}F-fluoride PET, and vascular calcification in atherosclerotic plaque: a dual-tracer PET/CT study. J Nucl Med 2011;52(7):1020–7.

34. Alavi A, Newberg AB, Souder E, et al. Quantitative analysis of PET and MRI data in normal aging and Alzheimer's disease: atrophy weighted total brain metabolism and absolute whole brain metabolism as reliable discriminators. J Nucl Med 1993;34(10):1681–7.

Can Vascular Wall 18F-FDG Uptake on PET Imaging Serve as a Biomarker of Vulnerable Atherosclerotic Plaque?

Wengen Chen, MD, PhD

KEYWORDS

• FDG PET/CT • Atherosclerosis • Biomarker

A vulnerable atherosclerotic plaque is defined functionally as a thrombosis-prone plaque that has a high probability of undergoing rapid progression. Morphologically, it typically has a necrotic lipid core with a thin fibrous cap and large amount of macrophages, without significant luminal narrowing caused by vascular wall remodeling. However, an advanced stable plaque usually has significant calcifications with luminal narrowing. Clinically, when a vulnerable plaque ruptures it can cause myocardial infarction, sudden cardiac death, or stroke if in the carotid artery. Current cardiovascular imaging modalities, such as coronary artery catheterization, CT angiography, and even nuclear myocardial perfusion studies, can only identify coronary artery luminal narrowing and its downstream flow-limiting functional consequence caused by advanced calcified plaques. None of these imaging techniques can identify non–flow-limiting vulnerable plaques. Hence, it is important to develop a noninvasive imaging technique that targets vulnerable plaques for diagnosis and treatment evaluation. 18F-fluorodeoxyglucose (FDG) imaging with PET likely provides the most promising tool for this purpose.

VASCULAR FDG UPTAKE AND PLAQUE INFLAMMATION

A vulnerable plaque is highly inflammatory and hence prone to rupture. FDG is a nonspecific tracer that also accumulates in inflammatory sites. It is common to see focal vascular FDG uptake in patients with an FDG PET/CT scan, which may represent a vulnerable plaque (Fig. 1). Intensity of vascular FDG uptake may represent severity of plaque inflammation. Animal studies have shown that FDG was taken up by macrophage-rich atherosclerotic lesions in the aortic arch, and there was a correlation between FDG accumulation in the plaque with local macrophage density.[1–4] In humans, accumulation of ^{3}H-deoxyglucose was seen in macrophage-rich areas of freshly isolated human carotid plaques,[5] along with a significant correlation between FDG-PET activity in carotid plaques and macrophage staining from the corresponding histologic sections of postendarterectomy samples.[6] Thus, vascular FDG uptake is linked to plaque macrophage density and hence plaque inflammation. An FDG-avid site could thus represent a highly

The author has nothing to disclose.
Department of Diagnostic Radiology and Nuclear Medicine, University of Maryland School of Medicine, 22 South Greene Street, Baltimore, MD 21201, USA
E-mail address: wchen5@umm.edu

PET Clin 6 (2011) 417–420
doi:10.1016/j.cpet.2011.08.004

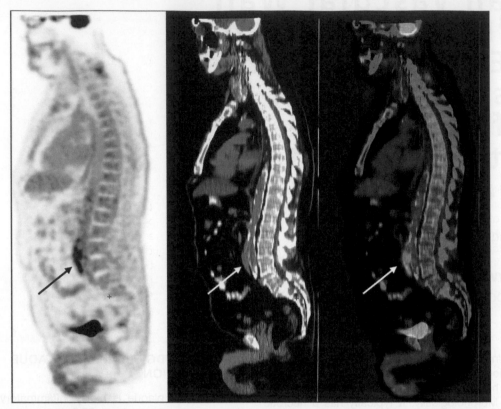

Fig. 1. FDG uptake (from *left to right*: PET, CT, and coregistered PET/CT imaging) in an abdominal aneurysm (*arrows*) related to atherosclerosis.

inflammatory, unstable plaque. However, it should be noted that severity of inflammation is not solely dependent on macrophage density. Macrophages can be either proinflammatory or antiinflammatory based on their activation pathways. Glycolysis is dominant in macrophages activated by classic pathway through proinflammatory cytokines, such as interferon-γ. Although with alternative activation pathway by antiinflammatory cytokines, such as interleukin-4 and -13, macrophages mainly use fatty acid oxidation as an energy source. In addition, other factors, such as peroxisome proliferators-activated receptors, which are expressed in plaque macrophages, regulate expression of genes involved in lipid metabolism, glucose homeostasis, and inflammatory response. Hence, plaque macrophage glucose use and inflammation is a dynamic and complicated process, and it is important to correlate vascular FDG uptake with plaque macrophage activations, in addition to density. It was found that acetylated low density lipoprotein (AcLDL) loading could significantly increase macrophage glucose consumption, probably through classic activation pathway (**Fig. 2**; Chen and colleagues unpublished data, 2009). Further studies are needed to elucidate

plaque macrophage activation pathway, inflammation, and FDG uptake on PET.

VASCULAR FDG UPTAKE AS A BIOMARKER OF VULNERABLE PLAQUE

To serve as a biomarker of vulnerable plaques, vascular FDG uptake should be (1) reproducible within a certain time period, (2) responsive to therapy, and (3) predictable to future cardiovascular

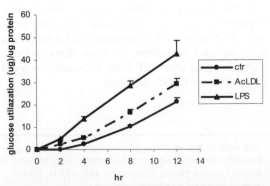

Fig. 2. AcLDL induces macrophage glucose in a time-dependent pattern. CTR, control; LPS, lipopolysaccharide.

events. A few retrospective studies showed that vascular FDG uptake was changeable in approximately 50% of sites within an interval of two PET scans ranging from 7 months to 5 years.[7–9] Two well-controlled studies found that vascular FDG uptake was stable at least within 14 days.[10,11] One prospective study showed that vascular FDG uptake was stable in 3 months.[12] Because vascular FDG uptake reproducibility (stability) is dependent on plaque inflammation, whereas atherosclerosis is a dynamic inflammatory disease, it is a dilemma to define the timing of vascular FDG uptake reproducibility, and more studies are needed.

A pilot prospective study regarding responsibility of vascular plaque FDG uptake to therapy showed that 3 months of simvastatin intervention significantly decreased FDG uptake in atherosclerotic plaques, whereas no change was noted in the control group with dietary management along.[12] Similarly, among patients undergoing a series of FDG PET/CT studies and atherogenic risk reduction by lifestyle intervention, vascular FDG uptake was shown to improve with risk factor modification. The magnitude of improvement in FDG uptake correlated with increasing plasma high-density lipoprotein level.[13] A recent prospective, randomized, open-label study showed that 6 months of atorvastatin, 20 mg but not 5 mg, significantly decreased FDG uptake in atherosclerotic lesions in the ascending aorta and femoral artery from baseline. The decreases in uptake were significantly correlated with reduction in LDL cholesterol.[14] An earlier animal study in rabbit showed that after 6 months of antiinflammation drug probucol intervention, vascular FDG uptake significantly decreased, which correlated with decrease in plaque macrophage density.[15] These results suggest that vascular plaque FDG uptake is responsive to therapy.

Studies have reported that the degree of inflammation in the culprit lesions could potentially be used to forecast future clinical events. Among patients with symptomatic carotid atherosclerosis and increased FDG accumulation, the subset of patients with intense FDG uptake suffered from subsequent death, recurrent nonfatal ipsilateral ischemic stroke, or restenosis after stenting.[16] A well controlled retrospective study compared cardiovascular events in two groups of stable oncology patients, with and without detectable large arterial wall FDG uptake.[17] Cardiovascular events were found to be significantly more frequent in the high-FDG uptake group compared with the low-FDG uptake group. A multivariate analysis showed that the extent of arterial FDG uptake was significantly related to the occurrence of a recent event. Patients with higher vascular FDG uptake had lower event-free survival than those with lower FDG activity.[18]

Although these studies are promising regarding the feasibility of vascular FDG uptake as a biomarker of vulnerable plaque, further prospective studies are needed to provide unequivocal data in terms of the reproducibility to time, responsibility to therapy, and predictability to cardiovascular event of vascular FDG uptake.

VISUALIZATION OF CORONARY ARTERY PLAQUES

Most of the studies regarding vascular FDG uptake on PET focused on large arteries (eg, aorta and carotid artery). Although atherosclerosis is a systemic vascular inflammatory disease and plaque information from large arteries could potentially represent those in the coronary arteries, there is clearly a clinical necessity to directly visualize coronary artery vulnerable plaques. Several factors limit direct visualization of coronary artery plaque: (1) small size of the coronary artery and plaques, (2) PET spatial resolution, (3) cardiac and respiratory motion during PET acquisition, and (4) background myocardial FDG uptake. All of these factors reduce the sensitivity of PET for coronary plaque identification. Nevertheless, some studies have clearly shown successful visualization of FDG uptake in coronary artery plaques.[19,20]

SUMMARY

Vulnerable atherosclerotic plaques, which are highly inflammatory but not flow limiting, account for most cardiovascular events, such as myocardial infarction, sudden cardiac death, and stroke. Current cardiovascular imaging modalities are based on anatomic detection of artery luminal narrowing, and thus are unable to detect vulnerable plaques. Hence, it is a laudable goal to develop noninvasive imaging techniques that target vulnerable plaques. Vascular wall FDG uptake has been shown to correlate with macrophage density and inflammatory status of plaques in animals and humans. Preliminary data have indicated the role of vascular FDG uptake as a biomarker of vulnerable plaque. Although it is still challenging, direct visualization of coronary artery plaques may become clinically feasible in the near future, with the development of a PET/CT technology that is optimized for cardiovascular imaging, along with progress in standardization of cardiac PET imaging protocol, such as dietary preparation, acquisition mode, acquisition time after the injection of the radiotracer, and cardiac gating.

REFERENCES

1. Ogawa M, Ishino S, Mukai T, et al. (18)F-FDG accumulation in atherosclerotic plaques: immunohistochemical and PET imaging study. J Nucl Med 2004;45:1245–50.
2. Tawakol A, Migrino RQ, Hoffmann U, et al. Noninvasive in vivo measurement of vascular inflammation with F-18 fluorodeoxyglucose positron emission tomography. J Nucl Cardiol 2005;12:294–301.
3. Zhang Z, Machac J, Helft G, et al. Non-invasive imaging of atherosclerotic plaque macrophage in a rabbit model with F-18 FDG PET: a histopathological correlation. BMC Nucl Med 2006; 6:3–10.
4. Davies JR, Izquierdo-Garcia D, Rudd JH, et al. FDG-PET can distinguish inflamed from non-inflamed plaque in an animal model of atherosclerosis. Int J Cardiovasc Imaging 2010;26:41–8.
5. Rudd JH, Warburton EA, Fryer TD, et al. Imaging atherosclerotic plaque inflammation with [18F]-fluorodeoxyglucose positron emission tomography. Circulation 2002;105:2708–11.
6. Tawakol A, Migrino RQ, Bashian GG, et al. In vivo 18F-fluorodeoxyglucose positron emission tomography imaging provides a noninvasive measure of carotid plaque inflammation in patients. J Am Coll Cardiol 2006;48:1818–24.
7. Ben-Haim S, Kupzov E, Tamir A, et al. Changing patterns of abnormal vascular wall F-18 fluorodeoxyglucose uptake on follow-up PET/CT studies. J Nucl Cardiol 2006;13:791–800.
8. Wassélius J, Larsson S, Jacobsson H. Time-to-time correlation of high-risk atherosclerotic lesions identified with [(18)F]-FDG-PET/CT. Ann Nucl Med 2009; 23:59–64.
9. Menezes LJ, Kayani I, Ben-Haim S, et al. What is the natural history of 18F-FDG uptake in arterial atheroma on PET/CT? implications for imaging the vulnerable plaque. Atherosclerosis 2010;211: 136–40.
10. Rudd JH, Myers KS, Bansilal S, et al. (18)Fluorodeoxyglucose positron emission tomography imaging of atherosclerotic plaque inflammation is highly reproducible: implications for atherosclerosis therapy trials. J Am Coll Cardiol 2007;50:892–6.
11. Rudd JH, Myers KS, Bansilal S, et al. Atherosclerosis inflammation imaging with 18F-FDG PET: carotid, iliac, and femoral uptake reproducibility, quantification methods, and recommendations. J Nucl Med 2008;49:871–8.
12. Tahara N, Kai H, Ishibashi M, et al. Simvastatin attenuates plaque inflammation: evaluation by fluorodeoxyglucose positron emission tomography. J Am Coll Cardiol 2006;48:1825–31.
13. Lee SJ, On YK, Lee EJ, et al. Reversal of vascular 18F-FDG uptake with plasma high-density lipoprotein elevation by atherogenic risk reduction. J Nucl Med 2008;49:1277–82.
14. Ishii H, Nishio M, Takahashi H, et al. Comparison of atorvastatin 5 and 20 mg/d for reducing F-18 fluorodeoxyglucose uptake in atherosclerotic plaques on positron emission tomography/computed tomography: a randomized, investigator-blinded, open-label, 6-month study in Japanese adults scheduled for percutaneous coronary intervention. Clin Ther 2010;32:2337–47.
15. Ogawa M, Magata Y, Kato T, et al. Application of 18F-FDG PET for monitoring the therapeutic effect of antiinflammatory drugs on stabilization of vulnerable atherosclerotic plaques. J Nucl Med 2006;47: 1845–50.
16. Arauz A, Hoyos L, Zenteno M, et al. Carotid plaque inflammation detected by 18F-fluorodeoxyglucose-positron emission tomography. Pilot study. Clin Neurol Neurosurg 2007;109:409–12.
17. Paulmier B, Duet M, Khayat R, et al. Arterial wall uptake of fluorodeoxyglucose on PET imaging in stable cancer disease patients indicates higher risk for cardiovascular events. J Nucl Cardiol 2008; 15:209–17.
18. Rominger A, Saam T, Wolpers S, et al. 18F-FDG PET/CT identifies patients at risk for future vascular events in an otherwise asymptomatic cohort with neoplastic disease. J Nucl Med 2009; 50:1611–20.
19. Alexanderson E, Slomka P, Cheng V, et al. Fusion of positron emission tomography and coronary computed tomographic angiography identifies fluorine 18 fluorodeoxyglucose uptake in the left main coronary artery soft plaque. J Nucl Cardiol 2008; 15:841–3.
20. Wykrzykowska J, Lehman S, Williams G, et al. Imaging of inflamed and vulnerable plaque in coronary arteries with 18F-FDG PET/CT inpatients with suppression of Myocardial uptake using a low-carbohydrate, high-fat preparation. J Nucl Med 2009;50:563–8.

Role of Global Disease Assessment by Combined PET-CT-MR Imaging in Examining Cardiovascular Disease

Babak Saboury, MD, MPH, Pouya Ziai, MD,
Abass Alavi, MD, PhD (Hon), DSc (Hon)*

KEYWORDS

- Atherosclerosis • ^{18}F-Fluorodeoxyglucose PET
- Cardiovascular disease • Global disease assessment
- Hybrid imaging

Atherosclerosis, the leading cause of cardiovascular events, starts in childhood and progresses over several decades.[1] As the degree of subclinical atherosclerosis increases, there is an increasing risk for cardiovascular events. The Framingham risk score (FRS) can estimate the 10-year risk of cardiovascular disease (CVD); however, there are significant limitations in using this method.[2–4] Other methods of predicting risk include structural imaging modalities such as angiography, ultrasonography, computed tomography (CT), or magnetic resonance (MR) imaging, which identify stenosis. However, the majority of cardiovascular events occur in subjects with less than 50% stenosis of their coronary arteries[5] and thus the identification of plaque that results in significant stenosis is not a useful strategy in predicting the future risk of cardiovascular events.[6] Plaque vulnerability is a multifactorial condition. Factors such as size and thickness of the fibrous cap and lipid core, as well as degree of plaque inflammation and molecular calcification, have all been shown to play potential roles in stability and vulnerability of the atherosclerotic plaque.[7–11] Therefore, an optimal strategy for reducing cardiovascular morbidity and mortality would be not only to detect atherosclerotic lesions but also to identify asymptomatic patients who are prone to plaque rupture and who would benefit the most from intensive, evidence-based medical interventions.[12,13] Modern molecular imaging techniques and those related to PET are able to identify and quantify inflammation, and thus have the potential to provide sufficient information about various stages of the atherosclerotic plaque. In particular, ^{18}F-fluorodeoxyglucose (FDG) PET/CT imaging is now considered a well-established noninvasive, accurate, and reproducible method in detecting and quantifying the process of cellular inflammation.[14–19]

^{18}F-FDG PET/CT can be useful in: (1) detection and quantification the degree and extent of atherosclerosis, (2) evaluation of the response to therapy, and (3) prognostication of CVD based on the intensity of the FDG uptake.

DETECTION AND QUANTIFICATION OF THE DEGREE AND EXTENT OF ATHEROSCLEROSIS
FDG and Inflammation

Glucose metabolism is one of the pivotal phenomena in the inflammatory process. In this

Two first authors contributed equally to this study.
Department of Radiology, School of Medicine, University of Pennsylvania, 3400 Spruce Street, Philadelphia, PA 19104, USA
* Corresponding author.
E-mail address: abass.alavi@uphs.upenn.edu

PET Clin 6 (2011) 421–429
doi:10.1016/j.cpet.2011.10.003

context, ^{18}F-FDG PET/CT, by measuring the metabolic rate of glucose metabolism, has been increasingly used to diagnose, characterize, and monitor disease activity and response to therapy in several inflammatory disorders, including sarcoidosis,[20] vasculitis,[21] inflammatory bowel disease,[22] rheumatoid arthritis,[23] and degenerative joint disease.[24] Accumulation of FDG in large vessel walls in the presence of an inflammatory disease was first reported as early as 1987 as a collateral report in Takayasu arteritis.[25] Later on, evaluating retroperitoneal malignancies, some other isolated accumulations of FDG in possible sites of inflammation (ie, in proximity to vascular graft) were also reported by Vesselle and Miraldi.[26] However, the first systematic study that linked FDG uptake in the large arteries to atherosclerosis was performed at the University of Pennsylvania. Retrospectively these investigators observed that 50% of their study population who had undergone FDG PET imaging for other purposes showed uptake of FDG in large vessels (abdominal aorta, iliac, and proximal femoral arteries) 1 hour after injection of the radiotracer.[19]

FDG and Atherosclerosis

The correlation between FDG uptake and atherosclerotic plaque inflammation has been addressed by several animal and human studies. Using a positron-sensitive fiber-optic probe, Lederman and colleagues[27] reported a 4.8-fold higher FDG accumulation in injured iliac artery (histologically confirmed to have a high density of macrophages) compared with the accumulation in normal iliac artery in New Zealand White rabbits. Similarly, in a study on a rabbit model, Tawakol and colleagues[28] showed that there is a significant correlation between the FDG uptake and macrophage-rich atherosclerotic plaque in aorta. FDG accumulation was related to vascular inflammation but not to the other components of the atherosclerotic plaque such as intimal thickening or smooth muscle cells. There are also other animal studies demonstrating the effectiveness of FDG PET in monitoring the therapeutic effects of low-cholesterol diet, statins, and anti-inflammatory drugs in atherosclerosis, which further suggest the capability of FDG in imaging and potentially quantifying plaque inflammation.[29–31]

In a study performed in 17 patients it was shown that FDG PET signal from the carotid plaques correlated consistently with macrophage staining from the corresponding histologic sections of postendarterectomy specimens. Recent transient ischemic attacks and severe carotid artery stenosis were associated with high FDG uptake in the lesion targeted for endarterectomy.[32] Using FDG PET, the prevalence of inflammation in carotid artery atherosclerosis was determined by Tahara and colleagues.[33] These investigators evaluated 100 subjects who underwent carotid artery ultrasonography for screening carotid atherosclerosis, and showed that 29% of patients with carotid atherosclerosis compared with 10.2% of patients without carotid atherosclerosis had documented inflammation (defined as standardized uptake value [SUV] $\geq$1.6). FDG has also been shown to significantly accumulate in nonculprit lesions. For example, Font and colleagues[34] reported the carotid accumulation of FDG not only in symptomatic stenotic lesions (with associated macrophage accumulation) but also in contralateral carotid with low to moderate stenosis, which suggests a potential role of nonstenotic lesions in future events, as discussed earlier.

FDG Uptake and Cardiovascular Risk Factors

A positive correlation has been found between arterial FDG uptake and various cardiovascular risk factors, and this suggests a potential role for FDG PET imaging in the detection and evaluation of atherosclerotic plaque inflammatory activity.

In a retrospective study performed at the University of Pennsylvania, there was shown to be an age-related vascular-wall FDG uptake in 50% of subjects older than 60 years in the abdominal aorta, and iliac and proximal femoral arteries.[19] Later on the same group reported the consistent correlation of age and hypercholesterolemia, the 2 most important CVD risk factors, with vascular wall FDG uptake in the large-vessel arteries.[18] The correlation between the degree of ^{18}F-FDG uptake and atherosclerosis risk factors has been described in several other reports, with one study noting hypertension also as a risk factor.[16,17] There is also a significant correlation between metabolic syndrome–related factors (abdominal obesity, fasting triglycerides, high-density lipoprotein (HDL) cholesterol, blood pressure and use of antihypertensive medications, hyperglycemia) and FDG uptake in carotid vessels.[35] Similarly, both impaired glucose tolerance and type 2 diabetes are reported to be associated with wall inflammation in the area of carotid atherosclerosis.[36]

Quantification of Atherosclerosis

Atherosclerosis is a systemic inflammatory disease that involves multiple vessel beds. Therefore, the presence and extension of plaque inflammation through the entire arterial tree can be considered as an important risk factor for future cardiovascular events. Because it is capable of quantifying the extent and degree of plaque inflammation, FDG PET can be used to predict the future risk of a plaque rupture and to monitor the response to therapy.

Different research groups have used different approaches to measure FDG uptake in atherosclerosis; however, the optimal method of FDG quantification is yet to be determined (Table 1). Rudd and colleagues[37] were among the first who attempted to quantify plaque inflammation. For quantitative analysis of PET images, they assigned a 3-dimensional volume of interest (VOI) to the area of stenosis of aorta on the contrast CT scan and then transferred it onto the coregistered PET images to produce mean FDG concentration values. The estimated net FDG uptake rate was then measured by dividing the mean decay-corrected plaque VOI FDG concentration by the integral of the decay-corrected input function (derived from venous plasma samples). Later on, Tatsumi and colleagues[17] used a visual grading score to evaluate the amount of FDG uptake semi-quantitatively: grade 1 slightly higher than blood pool and mediastinal uptake; grade 2 clearly seen and greater than grade 1 but lower than liver uptake; grade 3 equal to or greater than liver uptake. These investigators also used an SUV value corrected for lean body mass to increase the accuracy of their quantification method. Bural and colleagues[15] developed a new method of quantifying FDG uptake by combining SUV measurement on PET with volumetric data of the aortic wall provided by CT to measure the extent of atherosclerosis in the aorta. Multiplying the calculated wall volume for the mean SUVs, they obtained an atherosclerotic burden (AB) value for each segment of the aorta that contained both volumetric and metabolic information. Using this method they showed that arterial volume, mean SUVs, and AB increase with age both regionally (in each aortic segment) and in the whole aorta, as expected; however, the progression of AB was shown to be exponential compared with the linear progression of mean SUV and volume, demonstrating the stronger value of the combined

variables than that of the two taken separately. The reliability of the aforementioned method was also confirmed not only in the aorta but also in other large arteries (iliac and femoral arteries) by the same research group.[38] Moreover, by avoiding the influence of the calcification volume (metabolically inactive with no further uptake of FDG) on the whole aortic volume and multiplying this corrected net volume by the corresponding mean SUVs over each segment, they were able to measure the global metabolic activity of each segment of the aorta, which was thought to be a more accurate estimate of disease activity.[39] Tawakol and colleagues[40] used blood-normalized SUV known as tissue-to-background ratio (TBR) for FDG uptake measurement. For this, a region of interest was drawn around the artery on the image of every slice of the coregistered transaxial PET/CT scan, and the mean SUV was obtained subsequently; they then measured the SUV of the venous blood to obtain a background value for FDG uptake. Finally, by dividing carotid plaque SUV by venous blood SUV, TBR was calculated.

Reproducibility of FDG PET Atherosclerosis Imaging

Temporal reproducibility of FDG PET/CT in imaging atherosclerotic plaque must be established if PET imaging is to be useful in serial monitoring of treatment response for atherosclerosis. Prospectively and for the first time, Rudd and colleagues[41] reported the high interobserver and intraobserver reproducibility of FDG PET inflammation imaging in evaluating atherosclerosis of carotid and aortic arteries in 11 patients by doing the same study twice over a 2-week period (Fig. 1). Using the same method, they further reported the high amount of near-term reproducibility of FDG PET/CT plaque imaging not only in aorta but also in femoral and iliac arteries.[14] Rudd and colleagues also compared 2 methods of FDG uptake measurement and suggested that the mean and maximum TBR be used for

Table 1				
Quantification methods used by different research groups				
Year	**Authors**	**Vessel Studied**	**Population**	**Method**
2002	Rudd et al[37]	Carotid	28	FDG accumulation rate
2003	Tatsumi et al[17]	Aorta	85	Visual grading score
2006	Bural et al[15]	Aorta	18	Atherosclerotic burden (AB)
2006	Tawakol et al[40]	Carotid	17	Target to background ratio (TBR)
2008	Bural et al[38]	Aorta, iliac, femoral	149	Atherosclerotic burden (AB)
2009	Bural et al[39]	Aorta	12	Global metabolic activity (GMA)

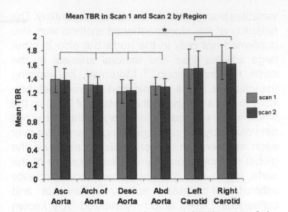

Fig. 1. Mean tissue-to-background (TBR) ratio of the first and second scan done 2 weeks apart. Error bars show standard deviation. Abd, abdominal; Asc, ascending; Desc, descending. (*From* Rudd JH, Myers KS, Bansilal S, et al. (18)Fluorodeoxyglucose positron emission tomography imaging of atherosclerotic plaque inflammation is highly reproducible: implications for atherosclerosis therapy trials. J Am Coll Cardiol 2007; 50(9);892–6; with permission.)

monitoring systemic arterial therapies and local, plaque-based therapy subsequently. In addition, Font and colleagues[34] evaluated patients before and 3 months following endarterectomy, and reported excellent FDG uptake reproducibility in the contralateral carotid arteries with less than 50% stenosis.

EVALUATION OF THE RESPONSE TO THERAPY

The reproducibility of FDG PET, as a noninvasive atherosclerotic plaque imaging technique, has made it an attractive modality to evaluate response to different cardiovascular drugs with anti-inflammatory properties (**Table 2**).[41] In 2006, Ogawa and colleagues[30] described the potential application of FDG PET/CT to assess the effectiveness of an antioxidant drug, probucol, on reducing atherosclerotic plaque vulnerability. Using myocardial infarction-prone Watanabe heritable hyperlipidemic rabbits, they reported

a progressive decrease in the amount of radioactivity of the aorta of the probucol group compared with the control group during the treatment (**Fig. 2**). The reduction of radioactivity was shown to be related to a significant reduction in macrophage density.

In a prospective, randomized, controlled study on 43 cancer patients with incidental finding of FDG uptake in aortic and carotid arteries, Tahara and colleagues[42] evaluated the effectiveness of FDG PET/CT in identifying the anti-inflammatory effect of simvastatin on the atherosclerotic plaque. This study showed that treatment by simvastatin was associated with a significant reduction in FDG uptake and SUVs of the plaque (**Fig. 3**). These investigators also showed that FDG PET/CT could identify plaque regression after only 3 months of statin therapy, which is much earlier than for any structural changes detected on MR imaging, which reportedly takes 12 months. Following this, another research group also reported the effectiveness of FDG PET/CT for evaluating the anti-inflammatory effect of another statin (atorvastatin) on atherosclerotic plaque. The study described a significant reduction in TBR in the ascending aorta and femoral artery following 6 months of treatment with 20 mg/d atorvastatin.[43] Furthermore, in a study on 49 patients with impaired glucose tolerance, Duivenvoorden and colleagues[44] compared the effect of pioglitazone versus glimepiride therapy on FDG accumulation, and reported a significant reduction of FDG uptake in the pioglitazone group. Lifestyle modification was also shown to be associated with the change of vascular FDG uptake. Using serial PET/CT scans, Lee and colleagues[45] reported a reduction of FDG accumulation in response to atherogenic risk reduction through lifestyle intervention (**Fig. 4**). This study showed that FDG uptake on follow-up PET/CT was significantly reversed with dietary modification, physical exercise, and weight reduction, and the magnitude of FDG uptake reduction was closely correlated with the amount of increase of HDL in the follow-up period.

Table 2
Interventions used by different research groups to evaluate treatment response

Year	Authors	Intervention	Population
2006	Ogawa et al[30]	Probucol	Hyperlipidemic rabbits
2006	Tahara et al[42]	Simvastatin	43 cancer patients
2008	Lee et al[45]	Life style modification	60 healthy adults
2010	Ishii et al[43]	Atorvastatin	30 PCI-scheduled patients
2010	Duivenvoorden and Fayad[44]	Pioglitazone	49 IGT patients

Abbreviations: IGT, impaired glucose tolerance; PCI, percutaneous coronary intervention.

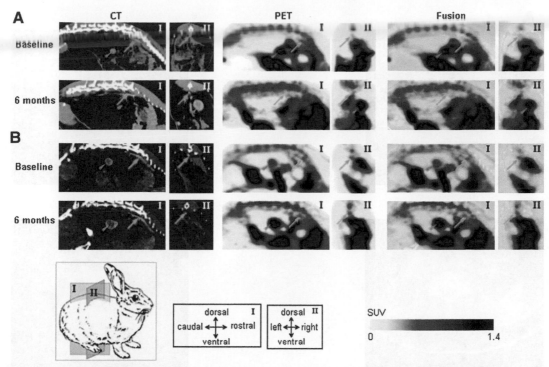

Fig. 2. Sagittal (I) and coronal (II) planes of PET, CT, and coregistered FDG-PET/CT images for probucol-treated (*A*) or control (*B*) rabbits before and after 6 months of therapy. Green arrows show aortas; pink arrowheads indicate kidneys. SUV, standardized uptake value. (*From* Ogawa M, Magata Y, Kato T, et al. Application of ¹⁸F-FDG PET for monitoring the therapeutic effect of antiinflammatory drugs on stabilization of vulnerable atherosclerotic plaques. J Nucl Med 2006;47(11):1845–50; with permission.)

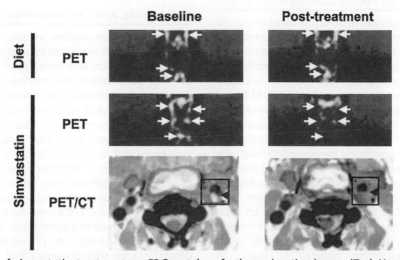

Fig. 3. Effects of simvastatin treatment on FDG uptake of atherosclerotic plaque. (*Top*) No effect of dietary management alone on FDG uptake (*arrows*) in the aortic arch and the carotid arteries. (*Middle*) Simvastatin is shown to decrease FDG. (*Bottom*) The superimposed images of FDG-PET and CT show disappearance of plaque FDG uptake (*arrowheads*) following 3 months of therapy with simvastatin. (*From* Tahara N, Kai H, Ishibashi M, et al. Simvastatin attenuates plaque inflammation: evaluation by fluorodeoxyglucose positron emission tomography. J Am Coll Cardiol 2006;48(9):1825–31; with permission.)

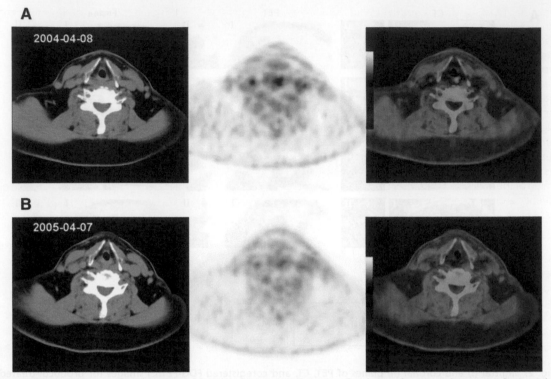

Fig. 4. FDG PET/CT images of 62-year-old male patient. (*A*) There is a focal site of increased FDG uptake in right common carotid artery in the initial scan. (*B*) One year later, carotid artery lesion is no longer visible following lifestyle modification. (*From* Lee SJ, On YK, Lee EJ, et al. Reversal of vascular ^{18}F-FDG uptake with plasma high-density lipoprotein elevation by atherogenic risk reduction. J Nucl Med 2008;49(8):1277–82; with permission.)

FDG AND PROGNOSTICATION OF CVD
FDG Uptake and Cardiovascular Structural Imaging Findings (as the Surrogates of CVD)

Vascular accumulation of FDG has been shown to be linked to some nonmetabolic characteristics of vulnerable atherosclerotic plaque measured by structural imaging techniques. In a study performed by Hyafil and colleagues,[46] using an iodine-based macrophage-specific contrast agent (N1177), it was shown that there is a significant correlation between the intensity of enhancement detected with CT and both FDG accumulation measured by PET and high macrophage density confirmed with histology. In a recent study, by comparing the plaque echolucency on carotid ultrasound (a feature of high lipid content) and inflammation rate measured by FDG PET, the same group showed that FDG PET can predict the future risk of cardiovascular events not only in symptomatic,[47] but also in asymptomatic patients.[48] Finally, in a prospective study performed on subjects with recent transient ischemic attack, those with microembolic signals on transcranial Doppler were shown to also have carotid plaques with a very high FDG uptake, demonstrating a strong association between embolic events distal to carotid stenosis and plaque inflammation.[49]

FDG Uptake and Cardiovascular Events

There are several studies relating vascular FDG uptake to both previous and subsequent cardiovascular events. Rudd and colleagues[37] were among the first to describe the relation between FDG uptake and cardiovascular events; they showed that FDG accumulation rate was significantly higher (27% more) in symptomatic lesions (angiographically demonstrated to be the "culprit" ones) than in contralateral, asymptomatic ones. Similar results have been also obtained by Davies and colleagues[50]; however, they observed a relatively high FDG uptake also in angiographically nonstenotic lesions located in the vascular territory responsible for the presenting symptoms. In another pilot study in 13 patients with previous symptomatic carotid plaque they observed that all restenosis, recurrences, or deaths occurred in subjects who had a high amount of carotid FDG accumulation (SUV$_{max}$ $\geq$2.7) during the 6 months of follow-up.[51] There was a significant correlation between the degree of stenosis detected by angiography and vascular FDG uptake. In a recent study, Paulmier and colleagues[52] showed that there is a higher rate of recent cardiovascular events in patients with higher vascular FDG uptake than in the low-uptake group. Of interest, the high FDG uptake in the arterial wall was seen only in patients who had cardiovascular events less than 6 months before or after PET imaging, confirming the hypothesis of significant correlation between plaque inflammation and acute event also in terms of time. Finally, the results of 2 more recent studies performed on asymptomatic patients also confirmed the high value of the arterial FDG uptake in predicting subsequent cardiovascular events.[53,54]

SUMMARY

Based what has been accomplished over the past decade, it is clear that FDG PET imaging in conjunction with CT and MR imaging increasingly will play a major role in assessing patients with suspected or proven atherosclerosis. Because the majority of the medical facilities around the world use PET and CT in combination regarding this very powerful modality, the benefits gained from such applications will be substantial. Such benefits include early diagnosis of this potentially fatal disorder, increasing the potential for a successful outcome by individualizing appropriate treatment for each patient, and developing newer and more effective therapeutic interventions for the future. It is speculated that the use of PET/CT and possibly PET/MR imaging will bring about a major revolution in the management of patients with atherosclerosis, which will reduce the degree and the extent of suffering of a large number of individuals around the globe from this potentially curable but devastating disorder.

REFERENCES

1. McGill HC Jr, McMahan CA, Herderick EE, et al. Effects of coronary heart disease risk factors on atherosclerosis of selected regions of the aorta and right coronary artery. PDAY Research Group. Pathobiological determinants of atherosclerosis in youth. Arterioscler Thromb Vasc Biol 2000;20(3): 830–45.

2. Greenland P, Smith SC Jr, Grundy SM. Improving coronary heart disease risk assessment in asymptomatic people: role of traditional risk factors and noninvasive cardiovascular tests. Circulation 2001; 104(15):1863–7.

3. Michos ED, Nasir K, Braunstein JB, et al. Framingham risk equation underestimates subclinical atherosclerosis risk in asymptomatic women. Atherosclerosis 2006;184(1):201–6.

4. Schlendorf KH, Nasir K, Blumenthal RS. Limitations of the Framingham risk score are now much clearer. Prev Med 2009;48(2):115–6.

5. Ambrose JA, Tannenbaum MA, Alexopoulos D, et al. Angiographic progression of coronary artery disease and the development of myocardial infarction. J Am Coll Cardiol 1988;12(1):56–62.

6. Pasterkamp G, Schoneveld AH, van der Wal AC, et al. Relation of arterial geometry to luminal narrowing and histologic markers for plaque vulnerability: the remodeling paradox. J Am Coll Cardiol 1998; 32(3):655–62.

7. Bluestein D, Alemu Y, Avrahami I, et al. Influence of microcalcifications on vulnerable plaque mechanics using FSI modeling. J Biomech 2008;41(5):1111–8.

8. Kolodgie FD, Burke AP, Farb A, et al. The thin-cap fibroatheroma: a type of vulnerable plaque: the major precursor lesion to acute coronary syndromes. Curr Opin Cardiol 2001;16(5):285–92.

9. Libby P, Ridker PM, Hansson GK. Progress and challenges in translating the biology of atherosclerosis. Nature 2011;473(7347):317–25.

10. Vengrenyuk Y, Carlier S, Xanthos S, et al. A hypothesis for vulnerable plaque rupture due to stress-induced debonding around cellular microcalcifications in thin fibrous caps. Proc Natl Acad Sci U S A 2006; 103(40):14678–83.

11. Virmani R, Burke AP, Farb A, et al. Pathology of the vulnerable plaque. J Am Coll Cardiol 2006; 47(Suppl 8):C13–8.

12. Greenland P, Abrams J, Aurigemma GP, et al. Prevention Conference V: beyond secondary prevention: identifying the high-risk patient for primary prevention: noninvasive tests of atherosclerotic burden: writing group III. Circulation 2000;101(1):E16–22.

13. Taylor AJ, Merz CN, Udelson JE. 34th Bethesda Conference: executive summary–can atherosclerosis imaging techniques improve the detection of patients at risk for ischemic heart disease? J Am Coll Cardiol 2003;41(11):1860–2.

14. Rudd JH, Myers KS, Bansilal S, et al. Atherosclerosis inflammation imaging with ^{18}F-FDG PET: carotid, iliac, and femoral uptake reproducibility, quantification methods, and recommendations. J Nucl Med 2008; 49(6):871–8.

15. Bural GG, Torigian DA, Chamroonrat W, et al. Quantitative assessment of the atherosclerotic burden of the aorta by combined FDG-PET and CT image analysis: a new concept. Nucl Med Biol 2006;33(8): 1037–43.

16. Ben-Haim S, Kupzov E, Tamir A, et al. Evaluation of ^{18}F-FDG uptake and arterial wall calcifications using ^{18}F-FDG PET/CT. J Nucl Med 2004;45(11):1816–21.

17. Tatsumi M, Cohade C, Nakamoto Y, et al. Fluorodeoxyglucose uptake in the aortic wall at PET/CT: possible finding for active atherosclerosis. Radiology 2003;229(3):831–7.

18. Yun M, Jang S, Cucchiara A, et al. [18]F FDG uptake in the large arteries: a correlation study with the atherogenic risk factors. Semin Nucl Med 2002;32(1):70–6.

19. Yun M, Yeh D, Araujo LI, et al. F-18 FDG uptake in the large arteries: a new observation. Clin Nucl Med 2001;26(4):314–9.

20. Brudin LH, Valind SO, Rhodes CG, et al. Fluorine-18 deoxyglucose uptake in sarcoidosis measured with positron emission tomography. Eur J Nucl Med 1994;21(4):297–305.

21. Otsuka H, Morita N, Yamashita K, et al. FDG-PET/CT for diagnosis and follow-up of vasculitis. J Med Invest 2007;54(3–4):345–9.

22. Basu S, Torigian D, Alavi A. The role of modern molecular imaging techniques in gastroenterology. Gastroenterology 2008;135(4):1055–61.

23. Vogel WV, van Riel PL, Oyen WJ. FDG-PET/CT can visualise the extent of inflammation in rheumatoid arthritis of the tarsus. Eur J Nucl Med Mol Imaging 2007;34(3):439.

24. Basu S, Zhuang H, Torigian DA, et al. Functional imaging of inflammatory diseases using nuclear medicine techniques. Semin Nucl Med 2009;39(2):124–45.

25. Theron J, Tyler JL. Takayasu's arteritis of the aortic arch: endovascular treatment and correlation with positron emission tomography. AJNR Am J Neuroradiol 1987;8(4):621–6.

26. Vesselle HJ, Miraldi FD. FDG PET of the retroperitoneum: normal anatomy, variants, pathologic conditions, and strategies to avoid diagnostic pitfalls. Radiographics 1998;18(4):805–23 [discussion: 823–4].

27. Lederman RJ, Raylman RR, Fisher SJ, et al. Detection of atherosclerosis using a novel positron-sensitive probe and 18-fluorodeoxyglucose (FDG). Nucl Med Commun 2001;22(7):747–53.

28. Tawakol A, Migrino RQ, Hoffmann U, et al. Noninvasive in vivo measurement of vascular inflammation with F-18 fluorodeoxyglucose positron emission tomography. J Nucl Cardiol 2005;12(3):294–301.

29. Davies JR, Izquierdo-Garcia D, Rudd JH, et al. FDG-PET can distinguish inflamed from non-inflamed plaque in an animal model of atherosclerosis. Int J Cardiovasc Imaging 2010;26(1):41–8.

30. Ogawa M, Magata Y, Kato T, et al. Application of ^{18}F-FDG PET for monitoring the therapeutic effect of antiinflammatory drugs on stabilization of vulnerable atherosclerotic plaques. J Nucl Med 2006;47(11):1845–50.

31. Worthley SG, Zhang ZY, Machac J, et al. In vivo non-invasive serial monitoring of FDG-PET progression and regression in a rabbit model of atherosclerosis. Int J Cardiovasc Imaging 2009;25(3):251–7.

32. Davies JR, Rudd JF, Fryer TD, et al. Targeting the vulnerable plaque: the evolving role of nuclear imaging. J Nucl Cardiol 2005;12(2):234–46.

33. Tahara N, Kai H, Nakaura H, et al. The prevalence of inflammation in carotid atherosclerosis: analysis with fluorodeoxyglucose-positron emission tomography. Eur Heart J 2007;28(18):2243–8.

34. Font MA, Fernandez A, Carvajal A, et al. Imaging of early inflammation in low-to-moderate carotid stenosis by 18-FDG-PET. Front Biosci 2009;14:3352–60.

35. Tahara N, Kai H, Yamagishi S, et al. Vascular inflammation evaluated by [^{18}F]-fluorodeoxyglucose positron emission tomog-raphy is associated with the metabolic syndrome. J Am Coll Cardiol 2007;49(14):1533–9.

36. Kim TN, Kim S, Yang SJ, et al. Vascular inflammation in patients with impaired glucose tolerance and type 2 diabetes: analysis with ^{18}F-fluorodeoxyglucose positron emission tomography. Circ Cardiovasc Imaging 2010;3(2):142–8.

37. Rudd JH, Warburton EA, Fryer TD, et al. Imaging atherosclerotic plaque inflammation with [^{18}F]-fluo-rodeoxyglucose positron emission tomography. Circulation 2002;105(23):2708–11.

38. Bural GG, Torigian DA, Chamroonrat W, et al. FDG-PET is an effective imaging modality to detect and quantify age-related atherosclerosis in large arteries. Eur J Nucl Med Mol Imaging 2008;35(3):562–9.

39. Bural GG, Torigian DA, Botvinick E, et al. A pilot study of changes in (18)F-FDG uptake, calcification and global metabolic activity of the aorta with aging. Hell J Nucl Med 2009;12(2):123–8.

40. Tawakol A, Migrino RQ, Bashian GG, et al. In vivo ^{18}F-fluorodeoxyglucose positron emission tomog-raphy imaging provides a noninvasive measure of carotid plaque inflammation in patients. J Am Coll Cardiol 2006;48(9):1818–24.

41. Rudd JH, Myers KS, Bansilal S, et al. (18)Fluoro-deoxyglucose positron emission tomography imaging of atherosclerotic plaque inflammation is highly reproducible: implications for atherosclerosis therapy trials. J Am Coll Cardiol 2007;50(9):892–6.

42. Tahara N, Kai H, Ishibashi M, et al. Simvastatin atten-uates plaque inflammation: evaluation by fluorodeox-yglucose positron emission tomography. J Am Coll Cardiol 2006;48(9):1825–31.

43. Ishii H, Nishio M, Takahashi H, et al. Comparison of atorvastatin 5 and 20 mg/d for reducing F-18 fluorodeoxyglucose uptake in atherosclerotic pla-ques on positron emission tomography/computed tomography: a randomized, investigator-blinded, open-label, 6-month study in Japanese adults scheduled for percutaneous coronary interven-tion. Clin Ther 2010;32(14):2337–47.

44. Duivenvoorden R, Fayad ZA. Utility of atheroscle-rosis imaging in the evaluation of high-density lipo-protein-raising therapies. Curr Atheroscler Rep 2011;13(3):277–84.

45. Lee SJ, On YK, Lee EJ, et al. Reversal of vascular ^{18}F-FDG uptake with plasma high-density lipoprotein elevation by atherogenic risk reduction. J Nucl Med 2008;49(8):1277–82.

46. Hyafil F, Cornily JC, Rudd JH, et al. Quantification of inflammation within rabbit atherosclerotic plaques using the macrophage-specific CT contrast agent N1177: a comparison with ^{18}F-FDG PET/CT and histology. J Nucl Med 2009;50(6):959–65.

47. Graebe M, Pedersen SF, Hojgaard L, et al. [18]FDG PET and ultrasound echolucency in carotid artery plaques. JACC Cardiovascular Imaging 2010;3(3):289–95.

48. Choi YS, Youn HJ, Chung WB, et al. Uptake of F-18 FDG and ultrasound analysis of carotid plaque. J Nucl Cardiol 2011;18(2):267–72.

49. Moustafa RR, Izquierdo-Garcia D, Fryer TD, et al. Carotid plaque inflammation is associated with cerebral microembolism in patients with recent transient ischemic attack or stroke: a pilot study. Circ Cardiovasc Imaging 2010;3(5):536–41.

50. Davies JR, Rudd JH, Fryer TD, et al. Identification of culprit lesions after transient ischemic attack by combined ^{18}F fluorodeoxyglucose positron-emission tomography and high-resolution magnetic resonance imaging. Stroke 2005;36(12):2642–7.

51. Arauz A, Hoyos L, Zenteno M, et al. Carotid plaque inflammation detected by ^{18}F-fluorodeoxyglucose-positron emission tomog-raphy. Pilot study. Clin Neurol Neurosurg 2007;109(5):409–12.

52. Paulmier B, Duet M, Khayat R, et al. Arterial wall uptake of fluorodeoxyglucose on PET imaging in stable cancer disease patients indicates higher risk for cardiovascular events. J Nucl Cardiol 2008; 15(2):209–17.

53. Grandpierre S, Desandes E, Meneroux B, et al. Arterial foci of F-18 fluorodeoxyglucose are associated with an enhanced risk of subsequent ischemic stroke in cancer patients: a case-control pilot study. Clin Nucl Med 2011;36(2):85–90.

54. Rominger A, Saam T, Wolpers S, et al. ^{18}F-FDG PET/CT identifies patients at risk for future vascular events in an otherwise asymptomatic cohort with neoplastic disease. J Nucl Med 2009;50(10):1611–20.

Relative Merits of Single-Photon Emission Computed Tomography and PET Perfusion Imaging: A Cardiologist's View

Abdulrahman Abdulbaki, MD[a], Kalgi Modi, MD[a],*,
Amol M. Takalkar, MD, MS[b,c]

KEYWORDS

• PET • SPECT • Coronary artery disease

Noninvasive imaging has gained an important role in the diagnostic and prognostic assessment of patients with known or suspected cardiovascular disease. Most of the diagnostic tests currently available are based on assessment of regional or global function under resting condition, stress condition, or both. Modalities include echocardiography, MR imaging, computed tomography (CT) angiography, and nuclear myocardial perfusion imaging (MPI) with either single-photon emission CT (SPECT) or PET.[1] The gold standard used for comparing sensitivity and specificity of the various noninvasive techniques for detecting coronary artery disease (CAD) remains invasive coronary angiography.

PET scan is a powerful, quantitative imaging modality that has been used for decades to noninvasively investigate cardiovascular biology and physiology. Because of limited availability, methodologic complexity, and high cost, it has long been seen as a research tool and as a reference method for validation of other diagnostic approaches. This perception, fortunately, has changed significantly within recent years. Evidence for diagnostic and prognostic usefulness of myocardial perfusion and viability assessment by PET is increasing. Some studies suggest overall cost-effectiveness of the technique despite higher costs, because unnecessary follow-up procedures can be avoided.

With the increased availability of PET scanners, the clinical use of PET myocardial imaging has grown. PET imaging has two major clinical cardiac applications: for an accurate and well-validated assessment of myocardial perfusion and blood flow in CAD or suspected CAD and its affect on ventricular function[2]; and for the assessment of metabolism and viability of myocardial tissue in the presence of systolic dysfunction and congestive heart failure caused by CAD.[1–5] In clinical cardiology, fluorodeoxyglucose (FDG) PET is considered the gold standard for assessment of myocardial perfusion and metabolism and provides the benchmark against which many new techniques are validated.[2,6–11]

Many technical and instrumental properties allow PET to operate as a highly accurate technique for cardiac applications. PET scan emitters work by releasing a positron from their core, which collides with an electron, thereby undergoing mutual annihilation and producing two photons

[a] Cardiology Division, Department of Internal Medicine, Louisiana State University Health Sciences Center–Shreveport, 1501 Kings Highway, Shreveport, LA 71103, USA
[b] Department of Radiology, Louisiana State University Health Sciences Center–Shreveport, 1501 Kings Highway, Shreveport, LA 71103, USA
[c] PET Imaging Center, Biomedical Research Foundation of Northwest Louisiana, LA, USA
* Corresponding author.
E-mail address: kmodi@lsuhsc.edu

PET Clin 6 (2011) 431–439
doi:10.1016/j.cpet.2011.09.002

that travel in exactly opposite directions (at an angle of 180 degrees). The characteristic of the two photons traveling in opposite directions provides the basic principle by which PET reaches higher spatial resolution, and is superior to other conventional nuclear techniques. The two photons hit the PET detector ring almost simultaneously (coincidence detection), which enables the technique to determine the collision site accurately.[8]

Spatial resolution of current PET devices reaches 4 mm in the center of the field of view compared with 10 to 12 mm for SPECT.[12] PET scans have higher detection sensitivity for the tracer concentration than CT and MR imaging.[8]

New detector materials and systems with reduced detection dead-time have recently been introduced, and three- rather than two-dimensional acquisitions are increasingly being used.[13–15] Image acquisition, which allows each event to be timed precisely according to electrocardiogram or breathing cycle, is widely available for clinical use.[15,16] At present, ^{13}N-NH3 and [82]rubidium (Rb) have US Food and Drug Administration approval for the assessment of myocardial perfusion, and ^{18}F-FDG for viability assessment.

ASSESSMENT OF MYOCARDIAL PERFUSION

The advantages of PET scan for assessment of myocardial perfusion are summarized in **Box 1**.[1]

Diagnosis of CAD

In a 2005 review of Machac,[5] eight studies that compared perfusion PET with coronary angiography observed a mean sensitivity of 93% and specificity of 92% for detection of significant CAD. Similarly, a meta-analysis by Nandalur and

colleagues[17] (**Fig. 1**) demonstrated a very high diagnostic accuracy from the available PET studies.

A limitation of SPECT MPI is the difficulty in distinguishing false-positive defects caused by attenuation artifacts from defects related to myocardial ischemia or scar. False-positive rate is higher than desirable for women and obese patients. Myocardial perfusion PET is considered to have superior diagnostic accuracy compared with the more widely available and more frequently used SPECT technique. The robust methods for attenuation correction with PET reduce the number of false-positive scans caused by attenuation artifacts, and specificity is increased. This is of particular importance in obese populations and women, where attenuation artifacts are frequent. Perfusion PET also tends to be more sensitive than SPECT, which can be explained by better spatial resolution and better tracer extraction at high flow, allowing for detection of more subtle perfusion abnormalities.

A direct comparison of SPECT with PET has shown significantly improved sensitivity, specificity, and normalcy rate in patients undergoing PET perfusion imaging.[18] An important finding in this study included a superior diagnostic performance of PET over SPECT when subanalyzed for gender and body mass index. Also importantly, the ability to identify multivessel ischemia with PET was significantly higher (74% vs 41%) than with SPECT perfusion imaging (**Fig. 2**).[18] These data suggest a substantially higher diagnostic accuracy of PET for the identification of CAD and for predicting the severity of the number of diseased vessels compared with SPECT.[1]

Prognosis of CAD

The greatest value of perfusion imaging is considered to be its potential to predict adverse cardiac

---

Box 1
Advantages of cardiac PET and PET-CT

Improved image quality

Higher spatial and contrast resolution

Accurate attenuation correction

Higher diagnostic accuracy

Excellent risk stratification

Rapid procedure

Rest and peak stress gating

Added information: blood flow, calcium, coronary CT

Data from Heller G, Calnon D, Dorbala S. Recent advances in cardiac PET and PET/CT myocardial perfusion imaging. J Nucl Cardiol 2009;16(6):962–9.

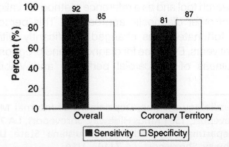

Diagnostic Accuracy of PET Perfusion: Meta Analysis of 19 Studies

Fig. 1. Metaanalysis of PET perfusion from 19 studies. (*Data from* Nandalur KR, Dwamena BA, Choudhri AF, et al. Diagnostic performance of positron emission tomography in the detection of coronary artery disease: a meta analysis. Acad Radiol 2008;15:444–51.)

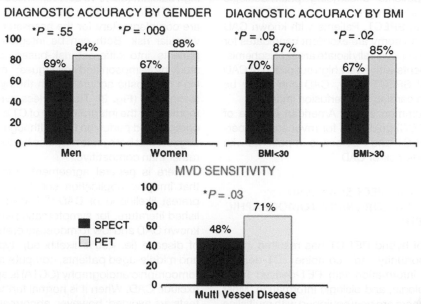

Fig. 2. Diagnostic accuracy: body mass index (BMI), gender influence, comparison of SPECT/PET disease severity. (*Data from* Bateman TM, Heller GV, McGhie AI, et al. Diagnostic accuracy of rest/stress ECG-gated Rb-82 myocardial perfusion PET: comparison with ECG-gated Tc-99m sestamibi SPECT. J Nucl Cardiol 2006;13:24–33.)

events. This incremental outcome information has been shown to be useful as a gatekeeper for invasive procedures and as a guide to appropriate therapy based on individual risk. Studies in very large patient groups have supported the incremental prognostic value for SPECT perfusion imaging. In one study, 685 patients were scanned with dipyridamole ^{82}Rb PET and follow-up was obtained over a mean of 41 months. The annual mortality rate was 0.9% for a normal scan and 4.3% for an abnormal scan.[19] In obese patients, a preferred target group for PET imaging and a group of individuals at higher risk, the annual total event rate was 11% with an abnormal scan and 1.5% with a normal scan.[20] Another recent study confirmed the prognostic value of dipyridamole ^{82}Rb PET in 1441 patients with suspected or known CAD, and it demonstrated an incremental value of stress left ventricular ejection fraction from gated PET.[21]

Flow Quantification

The ability to quantify myocardial blood flow (MBF) and coronary flow reserve (CFR) in absolute terms is another powerful feature of PET. Early studies showed adverse effects on CFR for multiple risk factors, such as hyperlipidemia, diabetes, or smoking, and supported the beneficial effects of

risk-factor modifications and novel medical therapies.[16] These studies have contributed to a paradigm shift in the perception of CAD, away from a pure macroscopic view of luminal stenoses and toward an emphasis on microcirculation and endothelial function. These are determinants of CFR and MBF and are key mediators of disease progression and risk. Several studies have suggested the prognostic value of quantitative PET measurements of MBF and CFR for progression toward clinically overt CAD.[22] Quantitative flow measurements may be useful and complementary to the current standard of visual and semiquantitative analysis. They may be useful for detection and evaluation of extensive multivessel CAD with balanced ischemia on qualitative images,[23] evaluation of the significance of a given lesion,[24] evaluation of collateral flow,[25] identification of endothelial dysfunction in preclinical disease, and reliable monitoring of therapeutic strategies.

The optimal patient selection for PET versus SPECT imaging is still emerging.[1] In patients with an equivocal SPECT study, the presence of CAD cannot be excluded without cardiac catheterization. These patients are excellent candidates for PET imaging to avoid invasive testing. Obese patients are also ideal candidates for PET imaging. Many laboratories recommend PET as the primary imaging modality in patients who weigh more than

250 lb. Consideration should be given for PET imaging in patients undergoing pharmacologic stress, because of higher accuracy of PET scans compared with SPECT. Patients with known CAD and complex anatomy are excellent candidates for PET imaging to specifically isolate areas of ischemia. Finally, in patients with a very high suspicion of CAD but a normal SPECT study, CAD can safely be excluded with cardiac PET perfusion imaging.[1]

Table 1 summarizes the American College of Cardiology (ACC) guidelines for myocardial reperfusion for SPECT and PET scans in patients with an intermediate risk of CAD.

HYBRID PET OR SPECT SCAN AND COMPUTERIZED CORONARY TOMOGRAPHIC ANGIOGRAPHY

The advent of hybrid PET-CT has resulted in the unique opportunity to combine CT-derived morphologic information with PET-derived functional, physiologic, and biologic information. Most PET-CT scanners are now equipped with multislice CT, allowing for CT measurement of coronary calcium or CT coronary angiography in addition to PET imaging procedures.

With the hybrid approach, Schenker and colleagues[26] observed an increasing prevalence of abnormal PET with increasing coronary calcium scores. Interestingly, abnormal perfusion was also found in 16% of patients with absent calcium. Among patients with normal PET MPI, the annualized event rate in patients with no calcium was lower than in those with high calcium (2.6% vs 12.3%, respectively). In patients with ischemia demonstrated on PET, the annualized event rate in those

with no calcium was also lower than in those with high calcium (8.2% vs 22.1%). These data suggest that CT calcium scoring and PET perfusion imaging are complementary for the assessment of cardiovascular risk. Both can be integrated to stratify patients into different risk-based categories. A study by Sampson and colleagues[27] demonstrated high diagnostic accuracy with the hybrid PET-CT technology (Fig. 3). There is less evidence at the moment for the integrated use of CT coronary angiography and perfusion PET, although initial studies suggest that both tests may also be complementary rather than competitive.

There is general agreement among clinicians that imaging application should depend on the pretest likelihood of CAD.[28] Based on the published literature, for symptomatic patients without known CAD and low to moderate pretest likelihood of disease (ie, <50% likelihood), typically young and middle-aged patients, computerized coronary tomographic angiography (CCTA) is appropriate to exclude CAD. When it is normal further diagnostic tests are avoided; however, abnormal or equivocal findings have to be confirmed or rejected by MPI or coronary angiography.[28]

MPI might be a better first-line test compared with CCTA in patients with higher pretest likelihood of disease (ie, >50% likelihood), characteristically those with known CAD or older age, likely to have extensive coronary artery calcium, and in patients with known or suspected microvascular endothelial dysfunction (eg, people with diabetes).[29,30] CCTA can be added in the presence of equivocal MPI findings suggestive of artifacts, microvascular disease, or multivessel disease. Also in these patients hybrid imaging improves

Table 1
ACC guidelines for myocardial reperfusion imaging for SPECT and PET

Indication	SPECT Class	PET Class
Identify extent, severity, and location of ischemia (SPECT protocols vary according to whether patient can exercise)	I	IIA
Repeat test 3–5 years after revascularization in selected high-risk asymptomatic patients (SPECT protocols vary according to whether patients can exercise)	IIa	
As initial test in patients who are considered to be at high risk (ie, patients with diabetes or those with >20% 10-year risk of a coronary disease event) (SPECT protocols vary according to whether patients can exercise)	IIa	
Myocardial perfusion PET when prior SPECT study has been found to be equivocal for diagnostic or risk-stratification purposes	NA	I

Data from Klocke FJ, Baird MG, Gateman TM, et al. ACC/AHA/ASNC guidelines for clinical use of cardiac radionuclide imaging: a report of the American College of Cardiology/American Heart Association Task Force on Practice Guidelines (ACC/AHA/ASNC Committee to Revise the 1995 Guidelines for the Clinical Use of Radionuclide Imaging). 2003 American College of Cardiology Web site. Available at: http://www.acc.org/qualityandscience/clinical/guidelines/radio/index.pdf. Accessed September 13, 2011.

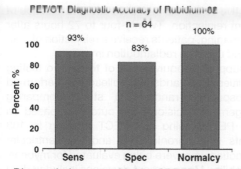

PET/CT. Diagnostic Accuracy of Rubidium-82

Diagnostic Accuracy: 99-99m SPECT vs Rb-82 PET
*P<.05

Fig. 3. Diagnostic accuracy of PET-CT hybrid imaging with rubidium-82. (*Data from* Sampson UK, Dorbala S, Limaye A, et al. Diagnostic accuracy of rubidium-82 myocardial perfusion imaging with hybrid positron emission tomography/computed tomography in the detection of coronary artery disease. J Am Coll Cardiol 2007;49:1052–8.)

diagnostic accuracy, providing a complete evaluation of hemodynamic relevance of coronary stenoses and assessment of viability in territories subtended by occluded arteries. The accurate spatial association of coronary stenoses and perfusion defects allows evaluation of hemodynamic properties of even fairly small coronary branches allowing for timely and appropriate treatment.[28] For asymptomatic patients with moderate pretest likelihood of disease, coronary artery calcium imaging is recommended as a reasonable choice for refining the risk stratification.[31] **Fig. 4** depicts a proposed clinical algorithm for the use of imaging in patients with chronic chest pain, based on a joint position statement by the European Association of Nuclear Medicine, the European Society of Cardiac Radiology, and the European Council of Nuclear Cardiology.[28]

HEART FAILURE

PET scan has several applications in the evaluation and treatment of ischemic and nonischemic heart failure. From a pathophysiologic viewpoint, there is generalized increased sympathetic activity in the hearts of patients with congestive heart failure. This contributes to the remodeling process. The myocardium of patients with systolic heart failure is characterized by a significant reduction of presynaptic norepinephrine uptake and increase in postsynaptic β-adrenoceptor density.[32] ^{123}I-MIBG imaging has demonstrated drug-induced changes in cardiac adrenergic activity. Treatment with angiotensin-converting enzyme inhibitors or angiotensin receptor blockers improved cardiac 123I-MIBG uptake without affecting plasma norepinephrine in patients with chronic heart failure. Similar improvements have been observed after treatment with β-blockers.[33]

Another application of PET scan in heart failure is to evaluate microvasculature dysfunction. Intramural coronary arterioles (<300 mm diameter) are primarily devoted to the regulation of MBF. There is no technique that enables direct visualization of coronary microcirculation in humans. Therefore, its assessment relies on the measurement of parameters that reflect its functional status, such as MBF and CFR. CFR is an integrated measure of flow through the large epicardial coronary arteries and the microcirculation. In the absence of obstructive stenoses on the epicardial arteries, a reduced

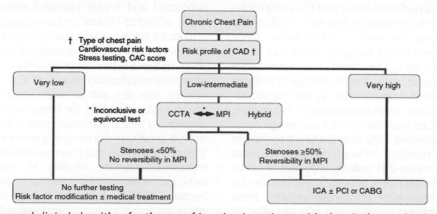

Fig. 4. A proposed clinical algorithm for the use of imaging in patients with chronic chest pain. CABG, coronary artery bypass grafting; ICA, invasive coronary angiography; PCI, percutaneous coronary intervention. (*Adapted from* Flotats A, Knuuti J, Gutberlet M, et al. Hybrid cardiac imaging: SPECT/CT and PET/CT. A joint position statement by the European Association of Nuclear Medicine (EANM), the European Society of Cardiac Radiology (ESCR) and the European Council of Nuclear Cardiology (ECNC). Eur J Nucl Med Mol Imaging 2011;38:201–12; with permission.)

CFR is a marker of coronary microvascular dysfunction. Although a single cut-off value of CFR (eg, 2) below which microvascular function is deemed abnormal would be useful clinically, it must be noted that in normal humans CFR varies according to age and gender.[34] Microvasculature function can be evaluated by measuring myocardial perfusion noninvasively with PET. Dysfunction of the coronary microcirculation can contribute to myocardial ischemia in the absence of epicardial coronary stenosis. The severity of coronary microvascular dysfunction is predictive of unfavorable outcome in patients with primary cardiomyopathies.[33,35] Measurement of absolute MBF in patients with cardiomyopathies may be of help clinically to identify at an early stage of the disease those patients who are at higher risk of evolving toward left ventricular dilatation and heart failure.[33,35] Studies have shown that PET can also be used to predict improvement of heart failure symptoms and improvement of exercise capacity.[36]

MYOCARDIAL VIABILITY

PET has perhaps been most thoroughly researched as a technique to assess myocardial viability to determine candidacy for a coronary revascularization procedure. For example, a patient with a severe stenosis identified by coronary angiography may not benefit from revascularization if the surrounding myocardium is nonviable. A fixed perfusion defect as imaged on SPECT scanning may suggest nonviable myocardium. However, a PET scan may reveal metabolically active myocardium, suggesting areas of "hibernating" myocardium that would indeed benefit from revascularization. The most common PET technique for this application consists of N-13 ammonia as a perfusion tracer and FDG as a metabolic marker of glucose use. A pattern FDG uptake in areas of hypoperfusion (referred to as "FDG/blood flow mismatch") suggests viable, but hibernating myocardium. The ultimate clinical validation of this diagnostic test is the percentage of patients who experience improvement in left ventricular dysfunction after revascularization of hibernating myocardium, as identified by PET scanning.

SPECT scanning may also be used to assess myocardial viability. Although initial myocardial uptake of thallium-201 reflects myocardial perfusion, redistribution after prolonged periods can be used as a marker of myocardial viability. Initial protocols required redistribution imaging after 24 to 72 hours. Although this technique was associated with a strong positive predictive value, there was a low negative predictive value (ie, 40% of patients without redistribution nevertheless showed clinical improvement after revascularization). The negative

predictive value has improved with the practice of thallium reinjection. Twenty-four to 72 hours after initial imaging, patients receive a reinjection of thallium and undergo redistribution imaging.

In support of equivalency of these two testing modalities, Beanlands and colleagues[3] performed a prospective randomized study comparing management decisions and outcomes based on either PET imaging or SPECT imaging in 103 patients with chronic CAD and left ventricular dysfunction who were being evaluated for myocardial viability. Management decisions included drug therapy or revascularization with either angioplasty or coronary artery bypass grafting. This study is unique in that the diagnostic performance of the two studies was tied to the actual patient outcomes. No difference in patient management or cardiac event-free survival was demonstrated between management based on the two imaging techniques. The authors concluded that either technique could be used for management of patients considered for revascularization with suspicion of jeopardized myocardium.

Therapeutic decision making is difficult in patients with advanced CAD and severe left ventricular dysfunction because revascularization has a high procedure-related risk. Viability testing has been developed to serve as a guide to the most appropriate therapy. **Fig. 5** demonstrates the superior assessment of myocardial viability compared with thallium viability. Several retrospective studies have focused on the outcome of patients with ischemic heart disease and ventricular dysfunction relative to their PET results and their treatment strategy. One such retrospective study has shown that patients who undergo a preoperative assessment of viability have a better in-hospital and 1-year outcome when a viability test is added to clinical and angiographic data.[37]

A recent meta-analysis summarized 10 studies in 1046 patients and found annualized mortality rates of 4% for those with viable myocardium who underwent revascularization versus 17% for those with viability who did not undergo revascularization. The mortality was 6% for those without viability undergoing revascularization versus 8% for those without viability not undergoing revascularization.[7] The recent STITCH trial also addressed the value of myocardial viability studies in patients with ischemic cardiomyopathy (left ventricular ejection fraction <35%) and showed that the presence of viable myocardium was associated with a greater likelihood of survival in patients with CAD and left ventricular dysfunction, but this relationship was not significant after adjustment for other baseline variables. The assessment of myocardial viability did not identify patients with a differential survival

Short Axis: Rest Thallium (Top) & FDG (Bottom)

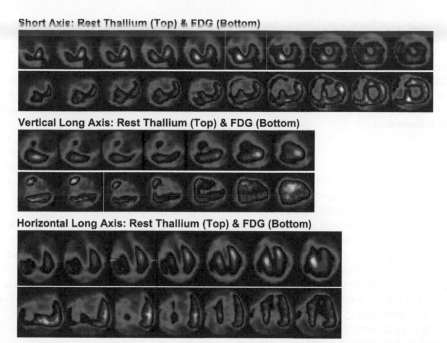

Vertical Long Axis: Rest Thallium (Top) & FDG (Bottom)

Horizontal Long Axis: Rest Thallium (Top) & FDG (Bottom)

Fig. 5. FDG-PET Myocardial Viability Study showing nonviable myocardium in a significant portion of the anterior and anteroseptal wall (compared with resting thallium perfusion) in a 46-year-old female patient with history of known CAD and cardiomyopathy, status post–cardiac catheterization and stent placement. Prior thallium study had reported 50% viability in the anteroseptal wall (based on which coronary artery bypass grafting would be an option for the patient). However, subsequent cardiac catheterization revealed akinesis in the anterior, apical, and mid-to-distal inferior walls with left ventricular dilatation and ejection fraction of approximately 15% to 20% with patent posterior descending artery (PDA) stents. Stress echo also confirmed akinesis in the anterior wall. FDG-PET myocardial viability study confirmed significant nonviable myocardium and it was decided not to proceed with coronary artery bypass grafting and revascularization.

benefit from coronary artery bypass grafting compared with medical therapy alone.[38]

The current ACC and American Heart Association guidelines recommend that PET imaging "appears to have slightly better overall accuracy for predicting recovery of regional function after revascularization in patients with left ventricular dysfunction than SPECT." However, the ACC[39] guidelines indicate that either PET or SPECT scans are Class I indications for predicting improvement in regional and global left ventricular function and natural history after revascularization, and thus do not indicate a clear preference for either PET or SPECT scans in this situation.

COST-EFFECTIVENESS CONSIDERATIONS

In cardiology, imaging options are extensive and often redundant. Because financial resources in health care are increasingly limited, the question of cost-effectiveness is crucial. False-positives may result in unnecessary subsequent diagnostic or therapeutic procedures, which carry additional costs and risks. A missed diagnosis caused by a false-negative test, however, may result in

preventable adverse events that could impair life duration and quality. Patterson and colleagues[40] compared cost-effectiveness of exercise electrocardiography, SPECT, PET, and invasive angiography to diagnose CAD. They observed that PET, despite the high cost of a single test, shows the lowest cost per effect in patients with a pretest likelihood of CAD less than 70%. This was attributed to its superior diagnostic accuracy and avoidance of false-positive and -negative studies. Only when the pretest likelihood was greater than 70% was direct angiography the most cost-effective approach. Merhige and colleagues[41] more recently compared the frequency of diagnostic arteriography, revascularization, costs, and 1-year clinical outcomes in 2159 patients studied with PET and a SPECT control group. They showed reduced use of downstream invasive procedures when using perfusion PET versus SPECT, which resulted in lower costs with comparable outcomes.

SUMMARY

Cardiac PET is a powerful, quantitative, noninvasive imaging technique that is increasingly penetrating clinical cardiology practices. For clinical assessment of myocardial perfusion and viability, evidence for diagnostic and prognostic usefulness is increasing and cost-effectiveness because of high accuracy despite high single-test costs is suggested. The advent of hybrid imaging enables routine combination of PET with CT-derived morphologic parameters.

REFERENCES

1. Heller G, Calnon D, Dorbala S. Recent advances in cardiac PET and PET/CT myocardial perfusion imaging. J Nucl Cardiol 2009;16(6):962–9.

2. Lalonde L, Ziadi MC, Beanlands R. Cardiac positron emission tomography: current clinical practice. Cardiol Clin 2009;27(2):237–55.

3. Beanlands R, Chow BJ, Dick A, et al. CCS/CAR/CANM/CNCS/CanSCMR joint position statement on advanced non-invasive cardiac imaging using positron emission tomography, magnetic resonance imaging and multi-detector computed tomographic angiography in the diagnosis and evaluation of ischemic heart disease abbreviated report. Can J Cardiol 2007;23:107–19.

4. Ziadi MC, Beanlands RS, deKemp RA, et al. Diagnosis and prognosis in cardiac disease using cardiac PET perfusion imaging. In: Zaret BL, Beller GA, editors. Clinical nuclear cardiology: state of the art and future directions. 4th edition, in press.

5. Machac J. Cardiac positron emission tomography imaging. Semin Nucl Med 2005;35:17–36.

6. Machac J, Bacharach S, Bateman T, et al. Positron emission tomography myocardial perfusion and glucose metabolism imaging. J Nucl Cardiol 2006;13:121–51.

7. Schinkel AF, Bax JJ, Poldermans D, et al. Hibernating myocardium: diagnosis and patient outcomes. Curr Probl Cardiol 2007;32:375–410.

8. Gaemperli O, Kaufmann PA. PET and PET/CT in cardiovascular disease. Ann N Y Acad Sci 2011; 1228:109–36.

9. Klein C, Nekolla SG, Bengel FM, et al. Assessment of myocardial viability with contrast-enhanced magnetic resonance imaging: comparison with positron emission tomography. Circulation 2002;105:162–7.

10. Schwitter J, DeMarco T, Kneifel S, et al. Magnetic resonance-based assessment of global coronary flow and flow reserve and its relation to left ventricular functional parameters: a comparison with positron emission tomography. Circulation 2000;101:2696–702.

11. Vogel R, Indermuhle A, Reinhardt J, et al. The quantification of absolute myocardial perfusion in humans by contrast echocardiography: algorithm and validation. J Am Coll Cardiol 2005;45:754–62.

12. Pichler BJ, Wehrl HF, Judenhofer MS. Latest advances in molecular imaging instrumentation. J Nucl Med 2008;49(Suppl 2):5S–23S.

13. Schepis T, Gaemperli O, Treyer V, et al. Absolute quantification of myocardial blood flow with 13Nammonia and 3-dimensional PET. J Nucl Med 2007;48: 1783–9.

14. Knesaurek K, Machac J, Krynyckyi BR, et al. Comparison of 2-dimensional and 3-dimensional 82Rb myocardial perfusion PET imaging. J Nucl Med 2003;44:1350–6.

15. Schwaiger M, Ziegler SI, Nekolla SG. PET/CT challenge for the noninvasive diagnosis of coronary artery disease. Eur J Radiol 2010;73:494–503.

16. Bengel FM, Higuchi T, Javadi MS, et al. Cardiac positron emission tomography. J Am Coll Cardiol 2009;54:1–15.

17. Nandalur KR, Dwamena BA, Choudhri AF, et al. Diagnostic performance of positron emission tomography in the detection of coronary artery disease: a meta analysis. Acad Radiol 2008;15:444–51.

18. Bateman TM, Heller GV, McGhie AI, et al. Diagnostic accuracy of rest/stress ECG-gated Rb-82 myocardial perfusion PET: comparison with ECG-gated Tc-99m sestamibi SPECT. J Nucl Cardiol 2006;13:24–33.

19. Marwick TH, Shan K, Patel S, et al. Incremental value of rubidium-82 positron emission tomography for prognostic assessment of known or suspected coronary artery disease. Am J Cardiol 1997;80:865–70.

20. Yoshinaga K, Chow BJ, Williams K, et al. What is the prognostic value of myocardial perfusion imaging using rubidium-82 positron emission tomography? J Am Coll Cardiol 2006;48:1029–39.

21. Lertsburapa K, Ahlberg AW, Bateman TM, et al. Independent and incremental prognostic value of left ventricular ejection fraction determined by stress gated rubidium 82 PET imaging in patients with known or suspected coronary artery disease. J Nucl Cardiol 2008;15:745–53.

22. Schindler TH, Nitzsche EU, Schelbert HR, et al. Positron emission tomography-measured abnormal responses of myocardial blood flow to sympathetic stimulation are associated with the risk of developing cardiovascular events. J Am Coll Cardiol 2005;45:1505–12.

23. Parkash R, deKemp RA, Ruddy TD, et al. Potential utility of rubidium 82 PET quantification in patients with 3-vessel coronary artery disease. J Nucl Cardiol 2004;11:440–9.

24. Muzik O, Duvernoy C, Beanlands RS, et al. Assessment of diagnostic performance of quantitative flow measurements in normal subjects and patients with angiographically documented coronary artery disease by means of nitrogen-13 ammonia and positron emission tomography. J Am Coll Cardiol 1998; 31:534–40.

25. Demer LL, Gould KL, Goldstein RA, et al. Noninvasive assessment of coronary collaterals in man by PET perfusion imaging. J Nucl Med 1990;31:259–70.

26. Schenker MP, Dorbala S, Hong EC, et al. Interrelation of coronary calcification, myocardial ischemia, and outcomes in patients with intermediate likelihood of coronary artery disease: a combined positron emission tomography/computed tomography study. Circulation 2008;117:1693–700.

27. Sampson UK, Dorbala S, Limaye A, et al. Diagnostic accuracy of rubidium-82 myocardial perfusion imaging with hybrid positron emission tomography/computed tomography in the detection of coronary artery disease. J Am Coll Cardiol 2007; 49:1052–8.

28. Flotats A, Knuuti J, Gutberlet M, et al. Hybrid cardiac imaging: SPECT/CT and PET/CT. A joint position statement by the European Association of Nuclear Medicine (EANM), the European Society of Cardiac Radiology (ESCR) and the European Council of Nuclear Cardiology (ECNC). Eur J Nucl Med Mol Imaging 2011;38:201–12.

29. Berman DS, Hachamovitch R, Shaw LJ, et al. Roles of nuclear cardiology, cardiac computed tomography, and cardiac magnetic resonance: assessment of patients with suspected coronary artery disease. J Nucl Med 2006;47:74–82.

30. Sato A, Nozato T, Hikita H, et al. Incremental value of combining 64-slice computed tomography angiography with stress nuclear myocardial perfusion imaging to improve noninvasive detection of coronary artery disease. J Nucl Cardiol 2010;17:19–26.

31. Greenland P, Bonow RO, Brundage BH, et al. ACCF/AHA 2007 clinical expert consensus document on coronary artery calcium scoring by computed tomography in global cardiovascular risk assessment and in evaluation of patients with chest pain: a report of the American College of Cardiology Foundation Clinical Expert Consensus Task Force (ACCF/AHA Writing Committee to Update the 2000 Expert Consensus Document on Electron Beam Computed Tomography). Circulation 2007;115:402–26.

32. Caldwell JH, Link JM, Levy WC, et al. Evidence for pre- to postsynaptic mismatch of the cardiac sympathetic nervous system in ischemic congestive heart failure. J Nucl Med 2008;49:234–41.

33. Camici PG. Advances in SPECT and PET for the management of heart failure. Heart 2010;96:1932–7.

34. Camici PG, Rimoldi OE. The clinical value of myocardial blood flow measurement. J Nucl Med 2009;50: 1076–87.

35. Shah P, Choi BG, Mazhari R. Positron emission tomography for the evaluation and treatment of cardiomyopathy. Ann N Y Acad Sci 2011;1228:137–49.

36. Di Carli MF, Asgarzadie F, Schelbert HR, et al. Quantitative relation between myocardial viability and improvement in heart failure symptoms after revascularization in patients with ischemic cardiomyopathy. Circulation 1995;92:3436–44.

37. Camici PG, Prasad SK, Rimoldi OE. Stunning, hibernation, and assessment of myocardial viability. Circulation 2008;117:103–14.

38. Bonow RO, Maurer G, Lee KL, et al. Myocardial viability and survival in ischemic left ventricular dysfunction. N Engl J Med 2011;364(17):1617–25.

39. Klocke FJ, Baird MG, Gateman TM, et al. ACC/AHA/ASNC guidelines for clinical use of cardiac radionuclide imaging: a report of the American College of Cardiology/American Heart Association Task Force on Practice Guidelines (ACC/AHA/ASNC Committee to Revise the 1995 Guidelines for the Clinical Use of Radionuclide Imaging). 2003 American College of Cardiology Web site. Available at: http://www.acc.org/qualityandscience/clinical/guidelines/radio/index.pdf. Accessed September 13, 2011.

40. Patterson RE, Eisner RL, Horowitz SF. Comparison of cost-effectiveness and utility of exercise ECG, single photon emission computed tomography, positron emission tomography, and coronary angiography for diagnosis of coronary artery disease. Circulation 1995;91:54–65.

41. Merhige ME, Breen WJ, Shelton V, et al. Impact of myocardial perfusion imaging with PET and (82)Rb on downstream invasive procedure utilization, costs, and outcomes in coronary disease management. J Nucl Med 2007;48:1069–76.

Cardiac CT Angiography: Protocols, Applications, and Limitations

Minh Lu, MD, Charles S. White, MD*

KEYWORDS

- Cardiac computed tomography • Coronary CT anatomy
- CT angiography • Calcium scoring • Coronary stent

Coronary artery disease (CAD) affects 17.6 million Americans and remains the most common cause of mortality, with 425,425 deaths in 2006.[1] The traditional management of patients presenting with acute chest pain involves history and physical, electrocardiography (ECG), and cardiac biomarkers. Imaging modalities including chest radiography and fluoroscopy, coronary angiography and cardiac catheterization, echocardiography, and nuclear medicine are routinely used to assess and diagnose cardiac disease. However, the emergence of multidetector computed tomography (MDCT), with robust spatial and temporal resolution as well as decreased image acquisition time, has enabled accurate visualization of the coronary tree and cardiac structures. For example, noncontrast material–enhanced assessment of coronary artery atherosclerotic plaques (CT calcium scoring) is used for cardiac risk stratification in asymptomatic patients and monitoring of medical (statin) therapy. In addition, contrast material–enhanced CT coronary angiography has become established as a valuable method for several clinical applications, including evaluation of coronary artery stenosis, coronary artery anomalies, coronary artery bypass patency, coronary artery stent patency, assessment of myocardial viability, pulmonary vein anatomy prior to ablation,

and preoperative planning. The versatility and availability of MDCT has contributed to the increasing use of cardiac CT as an alternative technique in noninvasive diagnostic cardiac imaging.

CARDIAC CT EVOLUTION

Cardiac CT scanning was introduced in the 1980s with electron-beam CT (EBCT) to quantify coronary artery calcium (CAC). The EBCT scanner lacked moving mechanical parts and used a rotating electron beam to produce x-rays. With no rotating components, image acquisition time was relatively short and temporal resolution was enhanced for better depiction of the coronary arteries, which are subject to motion artifact. However, EBCT had limited spatial resolution and commercial availability, and was supplanted by the development of newer and more versatile MDCT technologies. MDCT scanners with ECG synchronization have the ability to assess not only coronary artery calcification but also coronary artery stenosis and cardiac function, as well as to analyze atherosclerotic plaque.[2–5] The diagnostic accuracy of MDCT in CAD significantly improved with each subsequent scanner generation, as demonstrated with the emergence of 64-slice and, more recently, dual-source 256-slice and

The authors have nothing to disclose.
Department of Diagnostic Radiology and Nuclear Medicine, University of Maryland School of Medicine, 22 South Greene Street, Baltimore, MD 21201, USA
* Corresponding author.
E-mail address: cwhite@umm.edu

PET Clin 6 (2011) 441–452
doi:10.1016/j.cpet.2011.08.002

320-slice CT scanners. The now commonplace 64-detector-row MDCT scanner can complete coronary artery acquisition within 5 to 8 seconds with a spatial resolution of 0.5 to 0.6 mm and temporal resolution of 50 to 150 milliseconds,[6] whereas newer-generation MDCT scanners with extended z-axis coverage and faster gantry speeds reduce susceptibility to arrhythmia.[2,7,8] This review provides an overview of cardiac CT and highlights some of the indications for this rapidly evolving technology (**Table 1**).

MDCT Protocol

Many imaging protocols are in use for MDCT evaluation of coronary arteries. Image quality depends on optimizing various patient and scanner parameters for better temporal and spatial resolution. To obtain diagnostic-quality MDCT images and reduce motion artifacts, the heart rate should be maintained at 65 beats per minute or less. This pace is usually achieved with the administration of β-blockers prior to image acquisition. Patients with contraindications to β-blockers can be given calcium-channel blockers. Sublingual nitroglycerin, a coronary vasodilator, can be administered to optimize imaging. Once optimal heart rate is achieved, the patient is positioned in the scanner, and attached to ECG leads and an intravenous contrast injector. In prospective ECG gating, the x-ray beam is turned on during a select phase of the R-R cycle and turned off during the rest of the cycle; this is also referred to as a step-and-shoot nonhelical acquisition, as the table does not move during image acquisition. In retrospective ECG gating, the x-ray beam is turned on throughout the R-R interval and images are acquired continuously with table motion. The main advantage of prospective triggering is the lower radiation dose compared with retrospective ECG gating. To reduce radiation exposure for retrospective gating, tube current modulation is developed using higher tube current during the most important part of the R-R interval with lower tube current in the remaining cycle. Retrospective

ECG gating, typically using the 60% to 80% phases of the R-R interval, enables the acquisition of multiple time points to optimize coronary artery imaging. Volume data sets from retrospective ECG gating can also be used to evaluate cardiac function. Cardiac anatomy is best imaged during the diastolic rest phase of the cardiac cycle when the coronary arteries are least prone to cardiac motion. A nonionic iodine contrast agent is administered through an appropriately sized cannula inserted into an antecubital vein. A preliminary topogram is acquired to ensure appropriate alignment as well as to enable the patient to practice breath-holds. Scanning is timed with the arrival of contrast in the ascending aorta, and can be adjusted using a region of interest placed in the aorta or left ventricle and then set to a predefined signal threshold of 100 to 150 Hounsfield units (HU). Alternatively, a test bolus of a small amount of contrast can be injected, followed by a saline flush to determine transit time. Based on the clinical indication, a calcium scoring image is often obtained first. Scans are usually performed in the craniocaudal direction and extend from the carina to below the cardiac apex (**Fig. 1**A). In patients with coronary artery bypass grafts (CABG), the scan range is shifted superiorly to include the origins of the subclavian or internal mammary grafts (see **Fig. 1**B). Images are acquired with a single breath-hold during mid-inspiration to reduce heterogeneity of contrast in the right atrium. The total time in the scanner including setup and image acquisition is generally less than 15 minutes. Axial cardiac images are typically acquired in a limited field of view (FOV) to allow for better resolution in evaluating cardiac disease (**Fig. 2**). A wider FOV can be secondarily reconstructed to encompass the entire thorax. Images are further reconstructed using curved planar reformation, maximum intensity projection, and volume-rendering techniques (**Fig. 3**). Additional dose-reduction strategies can be achieved with iterative reconstruction techniques, with the potential for improved image quality relative to filtered back-projection techniques.

Table 1
Technical parameters in currently available cardiac CT

Resolution/Coverage	64-Slice (Multiple Vendors)	256-Slice (Philips)	320-Slice (Toshiba)	Dual-Source with 128 × 2-Slice (Siemens)
Temporal resolution (ms)	165–200	135	175	75
Spatial resolution (mm)	0.5–0.625	0.625	0.5	0.6
z-Axis coverage (mm)	32–40	80	160	38.4

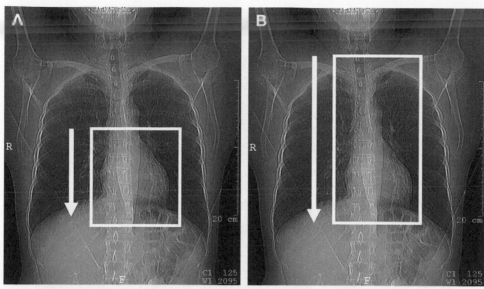

Fig. 1. (*A*) Anteroposterior topogram showing field of view required for dedicated coronary CTA (*arrow*). (*B*) Anteroposterior topogram showing field of view required for dedicated coronary CTA in patients with coronary bypass graft (CABG) (*arrow*).

CLINICAL APPLICATIONS
Coronary Angiography

Conventional coronary angiography is currently the gold standard and routine procedure for evaluating the extent of stenosis. However, increased economic burden, inconvenience to patients, and a small but definite risk of complications associated with invasive coronary angiography have driven investigators to seek alternative, noninvasive imaging techniques to visualize the coronary

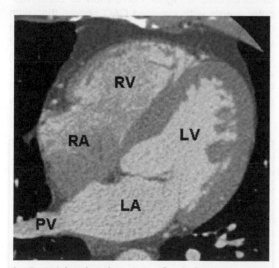

Fig. 2. Axial 4-chamber view of a dedicated coronary CTA. LA, left atrium; LV, left ventricle; PV, pulmonary vein; RA, right atrium; RV, right ventricle.

arteries.[9] In addition, conventional invasive angiography provides only 2-dimensional information on vessel lumen, which limits evaluation of the whole lumen of the diseased vessel wall. The development of ECG-synchronized MDCT led to the potential for noninvasive assessment and diagnosis of CAD through visualization of the coronary artery lumen, coronary atherosclerotic plaque, and coronary stenoses. Early investigations with 4-slice scanners reported sensitivity and specificity of 86% to 95% and 89% to 96%, respectively[10–12] in per-patient–based evaluation. However, limited spatial and temporal resolution as well as motion artifacts precluded imaging evaluation of stenoses in up to 32% of coronary arteries.[13] With the advent of 16-slice CT and improved collimation and gantry rotation time, sensitivity and specificity ranged from 85% to 100% and 86% to 98%, respectively, in per-patient–based evaluation.[14–19] The subsequent development of 64-slice MDCT with improved image quality and shorter acquisition time established its role in providing a rapid noninvasive assessment of the coronary arteries with sensitivity and specificity comparable with those of invasive coronary angiography. Recent studies suggest that 64-slice coronary CT angiography (CTA) is highly accurate for exclusion of significant coronary artery stenosis ($\geq$50% luminal narrowing), with a sensitivity range of 79% to 99% and specificity between 95% and 97%.[7,20–23] The high negative predictive value associated with 64-slice scanners (98%–99%) in comparison with

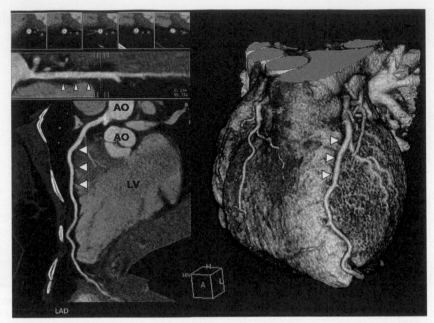

Fig. 3. Curved multiplanar reformation and volume-rendered views of the left anterior descending (LAD) artery in a normal patient (*arrowheads*). AO, aorta; LV, left ventricle.

invasive coronary angiography enables the exclusion of obstructive CAD following a normal CTA with a high degree of certainty,[24] obviating invasive cardiac catheterization, particularly in patients with low to intermediate risk of relevant stenoses.[25,26] According to recent guidelines, CTA is reasonable for assessment of obstructive stenoses in symptomatic patients. However, its use in asymptomatic persons as a screening test for atherosclerosis (noncalcific plaque) is not recommended.[13] In addition to its utility in evaluating CAD in symptomatic patients in the emergency department, CTA using appropriate protocols can reliably diagnose or exclude other noncardiac causes of chest pain, including pulmonary embolism and acute aortic dissection.[26,27]

Calcium Scoring

Noninvasive detection and quantification of coronary calcium using the Agatston scoring system for atherosclerotic disease has been well established.[28] Although EBCT has been shown to be effective in quantifying calcium scoring, spatial resolution is lower than that of MDCT. In addition, EBCT can be used only in sequential scanning mode, resulting in interscan variability. MDCT with spiral mode scanning and retrospective gating overcomes this limitation. However, for calcium scoring, prospective gating with sequential mode scanning is generally used for MDCT. Thus, MDCT is now used more widely for calcium

scoring, as EBCT is no longer widely available in the United States. CAC scoring has been used as an aid for stratifying cardiac risk.[29] The Agatston calcium score is based on density-weighted volume of plaques with an attenuation threshold of 130 HU. CAC scoring has been shown to be a strong predictor of cardiovascular events when compared with traditional risk factors, conventional angiography, and stress testing.[13] A prospective study by Detrano and colleagues[30] demonstrated a higher correlation of cardiovascular events with elevated CAC scores than with conventional cardiovascular risk factors. Recent studies have also concluded that the absence of coronary artery calcification (Agatston score 0) indicates a low risk (<1%) for subsequent cardiac events (**Table 2**).[7,31,32] CAC scoring studies often precede CTA for suspected CAD, and allow

Table 2 Calcium scoring	
Calcium Score	**Presence of Coronary Artery Disease (CAD)**
0	No evidence of CAD
1–10	Minimal evidence of CAD
11–100	Mild evidence of CAD
101–400	Moderate evidence of CAD
>400	Extensive evidence of CAD

patients to acclimate to the scanning and breath-hold procedures. These scans also aid technologists in identifying anatomic landmarks to determine the z-axis extent of the scan. Current American College of Cardiology and American Heart Association guidelines state that asymptomatic patients with an intermediate Framingham Risk Score may be reasonable candidates for CAC scoring as a potential means of modifying risk prediction and altering therapy (**Fig. 4A, B**).[33] Calcium scoring is generally not indicated for asymptomatic patients at high or low risk for CAD, because it does not change medical management in these patients.[34]

Left Ventricular Function

Accurate assessment of left ventricular (LV) function has both prognostic and therapeutic value in patients with coronary disease.[34,35] Retrospective contrast-enhanced ECG-gated MDCT enables the acquisition of data within a cardiac cycle, which can be reformatted and used to determine LV volume and global function. Although MDCT is not the primary modality for functional analysis, it provides additional useful information in patients undergoing MDCT coronary angiography for detection of coronary artery obstruction, without the need for further imaging studies or additional radiation exposure. Cine magnetic resonance (MR) imaging is currently regarded as the gold standard for the assessment of global and regional cardiac function. Early evaluation of the clinical utility of MDCT in assessing LV volume resulted in an underestimation of both end-diastolic and end-systolic volumes when compared with MR,[36] mainly because of the limited temporal resolution of earlier scanners. Further improvements in temporal resolution with newer MDCT scanners may facilitate assessment of cardiac function.

EVALUATION OF CABG

Conventional angiography remains the gold standard in evaluating the patency of coronary bypass grafts; however, in recent years improvements in MDCT technology have enabled accurate and noninvasive visualization of grafts. Several studies have explored the diagnostic potential of various scanner generations in the evaluation of CABG patency and stenosis.[37–39] The introduction of 64-slice MDCT scanners, with high spatial and temporal resolution, enabled detection of stenoses of coronary arteries and grafts with submillimeter collimation during a single breath-hold.[40] Interactive 3-dimensional (3D) multiplanar software now allows detailed depiction of arterial and venous bypass grafts and native coronary arteries, including the degree of stenosis caused by coronary plaques (**Fig. 5A–D**). Recent literature on 64-slice CT reports sensitivity and specificity ranges of 93.3% to 100% and 91.4% to 100%, respectively, in assessing CABG occlusion and significant stenosis ($\geq$50%).[41–45]

Liu and colleagues[46] evaluated the diagnostic accuracy of 64-slice CTA in 228 patients after CABG. The sensitivity, specificity, positive and negative predictive values, and accuracy for detecting graft stenosis were 93%, 98%, 93%, 98%, and 97%, respectively. For graft occlusion the comparative values were 96.4%, 98.1%, 96.4%, 98.1%, and 97.6%, respectively.

Evaluation of Stents

Cardiac CTA is limited in its ability to evaluate stent patency in coronary arteries. The diagnostic

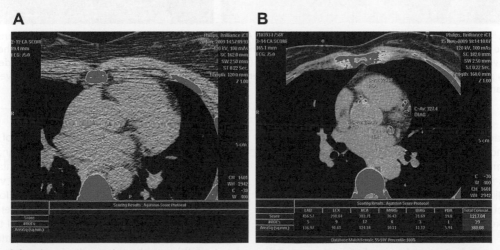

Fig. 4. (*A*) Calcium scoring by Agatston method = 0 in a 43-year-old woman presenting with chest pain. (*B*) Calcium scoring by Agatston method = 1217 in a 56-year-old woman presenting with chest pain.

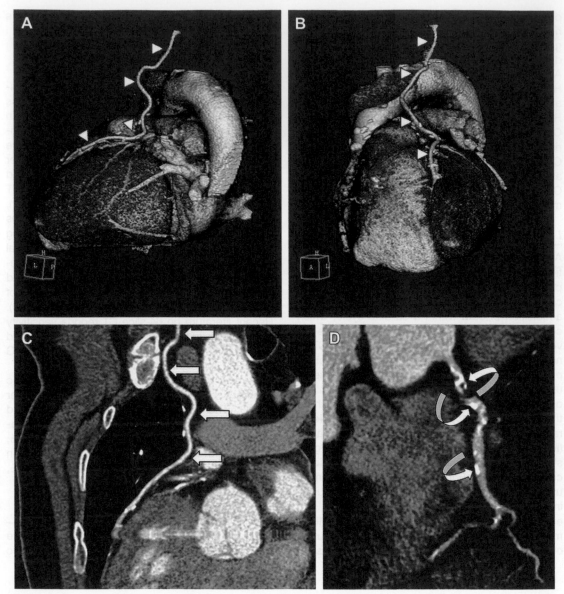

Fig. 5. A 60-year-old man who underwent cardiac CTA to evaluate for CABG patency. (*A, B*) 3-dimensional volume-rendered images show the left internal mammary artery (LIMA) (*arrowheads*) is attached to the LAD artery with multiple surgical clips adjacent to the artery. (*C*) Curved multiplanar reformation (MPR) image demonstrates patency of the LIMA (*arrows*). (*D*) Extensive eccentric calcified plaques along the wall of the native right coronary artery (*curved arrows*).

accuracy of MDCT in evaluating stent patency depends on various factors, including stent diameter, material, and design.[47] The degree of artifact varies with the type of stent material and design. Metallic struts in stents can create a blooming artifact, which can result in the appearance of a thicker strut and underestimation of lumen diameter.[48] Multiplanar and cross-sectional reformatted images are used to visualize and accurately assess stent patency, restenosis, or neointimal hyperplasia. In addition, characterization of contrast enhancement patterns is vital in the analysis of stent patency (**Fig. 6**). Coronary stents are considered occluded when no contrast is visible inside the stent lumen, with decreased or loss of distal runoff, indicating significant restenosis. Visualization of contrast in the vessel distal to the stent alone does not necessarily indicate patency, because this may be the result of retrograde filling of the vessels.[48]

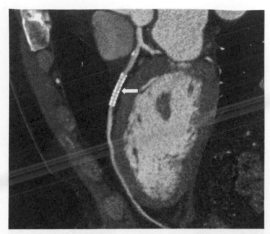

Fig. 6. A 60-year-old man who underwent cardiac CTA to evaluate stent patency in the LAD artery. Curved MPR image of the LAD artery demonstrates stent patency (*arrow*).

Assessment of Myocardial Viability

Coronary revascularization by percutaneous coronary intervention (PCI) in patients with acute myocardial infarction may improve survival with the identification and restoration of viable myocardium. The evaluation of myocardial viability using contrast-enhanced MR imaging has been well established. However, recent preliminary studies have demonstrated the potential of cardiac MDCT in assessing myocardial perfusion as an alternative technique.[49,50] Habis and colleagues[51] performed cardiac CT imaging immediately after coronary angiography without contrast reinjection and demonstrated a promising technique in early assessment of myocardial viability. Furthermore, myocardial hyperenhancement patterns may facilitate postinfarction therapeutic strategies. Further studies are needed to define the role of cardiac CT for myocardial viability assessment.

Venous Mapping for Atrial Fibrillation

Atrial fibrillation is the most common supraventricular arrhythmia. Ectopic arrhythmic foci originating within the pulmonary veins are a cause of both paroxysmal and persistent atrial fibrillation.[52] Radiofrequency catheter ablation (RFCA) of the distal pulmonary veins and posterior left atrium is effective as a treatment for paroxysmal atrial fibrillation in patients with refractory atrial fibrillation or resistant to pharmacologic therapy or cardioversion.[53] More recently, successful RFCA of atrial fibrillation has been aided by precise 3D anatomic mapping of the pulmonary vein using MDCT before the procedure. Multidetector CT of the pulmonary veins provides important anatomic information including the number, location, size, and orientation of pulmonary veins and their ostial branches noninvasively. Preprocedural mapping has been shown to decrease radiofrequency ablation procedure time.

CORONARY CT ANATOMY

Accurate evaluation of the coronary arteries requires knowledge of their origin and course. Initial assessment involves using the axial imaging data with the heart in an oblique plane. Postprocessed images, including short-axis views, curvilinear reformations, long-axis extended views of the lumen, and 3D surface-shaded volume-rendered images, are also used to analyze the coronary arteries. There are 3 sinuses of Valsalva in the ascending aorta, including the left (from which the left main coronary artery originates) (**Fig. 7**), the right (which gives rise to the right coronary artery), and the posterior or noncoronary sinus. The left and right coronary arteries may appear at different axial levels.

Left Main and Left Anterior Coronary Artery

The left main (LM) coronary artery arises from the left sinus of Valsalva and courses behind the main pulmonary artery, eventually bifurcating into the left anterior descending (LAD) and left circumflex (LCX) arteries (**Fig. 8**). A middle branch between the LAD and LCX known as the ramus intermedius may also occasionally arise from the LM artery. The LAD artery traverses anteriorly and inferiorly in the anterior interventricular groove toward the apex, giving rise to septal and diagonal

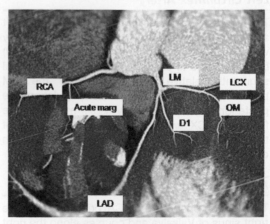

Fig. 7. A 46-year-old woman who presented with chest pain. Curved MPR image of the RCA and LM with branches. Acute marg, acute marginal branch; D1, diagonal branch; LAD, left anterior descending; LCX, left circumflex; LM, left main; OM, obtuse marginal branch; RCA, right coronary artery.

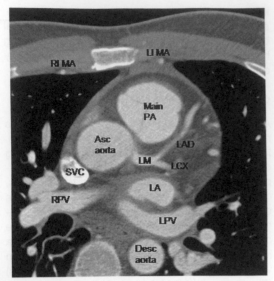

Fig. 8. A 25-year-old man with history of nonischemic cardiomyopathy who presented for planned insertion of an implantable cardioverter-defibrillator. Prospective electrocardiography (ECG)-gated axial images of the heart were obtained. Asc aorta, ascending aorta; Desc aorta, descending aorta; LA, left atrium; LAD, left anterior descending; LCX, left circumflex; LIMA, left internal mammary artery; LM, left main; LPV, left pulmonary vein; Main PA, main pulmonary artery; RIMA, right internal mammary artery; RPV, right pulmonary vein; SVC, superior vena cava.

branches (**Fig. 9**).[54] The diagonal branches course downward to supply the anterolateral free wall of the left ventricle while septal branches supply the anterior two-thirds of the interventricular septum.

Left Circumflex Artery

The LCX artery courses left and inferiorly in the left atrioventricular groove (**Fig. 10**). The LCX artery variably gives rise to 3 obtuse marginal (OM) branches, and is divided into proximal and distal segments relative to the origin of the OM branches.[54] In about 10% of the population, the posterior descending artery (PDA) may originate from the LCX artery as it reaches the crux of the heart, resulting in left coronary circulation dominance.

Right Coronary Artery

The right coronary artery (RCA) originates from the right sinus of Valsalva and courses along the right atrioventricular groove curving posteriorly (**Fig. 11**). The RCA is divided into proximal, mid, and distal segments. The proximal segment of the RCA (15–25 mm) runs along a horizontal course, is often seen on horizontal sections, and

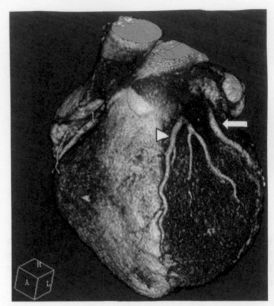

Fig. 9. Volume-rendered image of the heart showing LAD (*arrowhead*) and LCX (*arrow*) arteries.

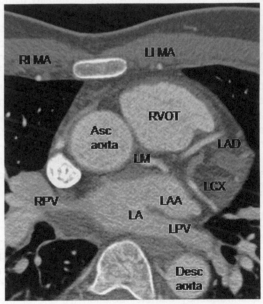

Fig. 10. A 40-year-old man with history of hypercholesterolemia who presented with chest pain. Prospective ECG-gated axial images of the heart were obtained. Asc aorta, ascending aorta; Desc aorta, descending aorta; LA, left atrium; LAA, left atrial appendage; LAD, left anterior descending; LCX, left circumflex; LIMA, left internal mammary artery; LM, left main; LPV, left pulmonary vein; RIMA, right internal mammary artery; RPV, right pulmonary vein; RVOT, right ventricular outflow tract.

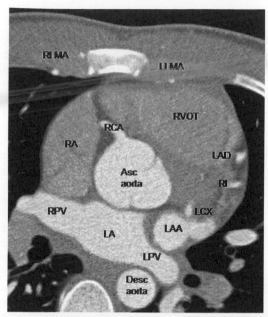

Fig. 11. An 18-year-old man who presented with chest pain. Prospective ECG-gated axial images of the heart were obtained. Asc aorta, ascending aorta; Desc aorta, descending aorta; LA, left atrium; LAA, left atrial appendage; LAD, left anterior descending; LCX, left circumflex; LIMA, left internal mammary artery; LPV, left pulmonary vein; RA, right atrium; RCA, right coronary artery; RI, ramus intermedius; RIMA, right internal mammary artery; RPV, right pulmonary vein; RVOT, right ventricular outflow tract.

extends from the origin to the acute marginal branch. The conus and sinoatrial branches arise from the proximal portion.[55] The mid to distal portions of the RCA extend from acute marginal origin to the horizontal segment along the right atrioventricular sulcus. The PDA originates from the RCA in 85% of the population and courses along the posterior interventricular groove.

Coronary Anomalies

Congenital anomalies of the coronary arteries are uncommon, and may be found incidentally in 0.3% to 1% of healthy individuals[56] during coronary angiography or CT. Certain coronary artery anomalies are clinically significant depending on the origin, course, and termination of the anomalous vessel, and may be associated with associated with sudden death, syncope, other congenital heart disease, or anginal syndromes. There are several types of coronary artery anomaly, with the wrong sinus coronary artery origin being the most frequent occurrence: specifically, anomalous origin of either the LCA or the RCA from the pulmonary artery, or an anomalous

course between the pulmonary artery and the aorta (interarterial) of either the RCA arising from the left sinus of Valsalva or the LCA arising from the right sinus of Valsalva.[57] Accurate recognition and documentation of coronary artery anomalies are essential in determining the significance of such findings and avoiding complications.

INDICATIONS FOR CARDIAC CT

Cardiac CT has emerged as a robust noninvasive modality in the evaluation patients with suspected CAD. Appropriate guidelines are continually being developed for the clinical application of cardiac CT. Current appropriate indications for CTA include[55]:

- Chest pain with intermediate pretest probability of CAD (uninterpretable ECG or patient unable to exercise, uninterpretable or equivocal stress test, or suspected coronary anomalies)
- Acute coronary syndrome with intermediate pretest probability of CAD (no ECG changes and negative serial enzymes negative)
- Evaluation of bypass grafts and coronary anatomy
- Evaluation of complex congenital heart disease (anomalies of coronary circulation, great vessels, and cardiac chambers and valves)
- Evaluation of cardiac masses or pericardial conditions in patients with technically limited images from echocardiography, MR imaging, or transesophageal echocardiography
- Evaluation of pulmonary vein anatomy before radiofrequency ablation, coronary vein mapping before biventricular pacemaker implantation, and coronary arteries in patients with new-onset heart failure
- Evaluation of suspected aortic dissection, aortic aneurysm, or pulmonary embolism.

Further improvements in spatial and temporal resolution, dual-source CT, and radiation dose reduction with evidence-based guidelines may expand the utility of coronary CTA to assess not only coronary and cardiac anatomy but also cardiac perfusion and viability in a single scan.

SUMMARY

Recent advances in multidetector CT, with submillimeter spatial resolution, improved temporal resolution, and ECG gating, make it possible to image and accurately characterize the coronary arteries. Cardiac CT offers the ability to noninvasively assess cardiovascular anatomy, including coronary arteries, bypass grafts and stents, my-ocardium, pericardium, and cardiac function. A growing body of literature supports the prognostic value of coronary CTA. This review provides an overview of clinical applications of cardiac CT, protocols used in performing such a scan, its limitations, and its future developments.

REFERENCES

1. Lloyd-Jones D, Adams R, Brown T, et al. Heart disease and stroke statistics—2010 update: a report from the American Heart Association Statistics Committee and Stroke Statistics Subcommittee. Circulation 2010;121:e260.
2. Ohnesorge B, Flohr T, Becker C, et al. Cardiac imaging by means of electrocardiographically gated multisection spiral CT: initial experience. Radiology 2000;217:564–71.
3. Kopp AF, Ohnesorge B, Becker C, et al. Reproducibility and accuracy of coronary calcium measurements with multi-detector row versus electron-beam CT. Radiology 2002;225:113–9.
4. Achenbach S, Ulzheimer S, Baum U, et al. Noninvasive coronary angiography by retrospectively ECG-gated multislice spiral CT. Circulation 2000;102:2823–8.
5. Juergens KU, Grude M, Fallenberg EM, et al. Using ECG-gated multidetector CT to evaluate global left ventricular myocardial function in patients with coronary artery disease. AJR Am J Roentgenol 2002;179:1545–50.
6. Hamon M, Morello R, Riddell JW. Coronary arteries: diagnostic performance of 16-versus 64-section spiral CT compared with invasive coronary angiography meta-analysis. Radiology 2007;245:720–31.
7. Raff GL, Gallagher MJ, O'Neill WW, et al. Diagnostic accuracy of noninvasive coronary angiography using 64-slice spiral computed tomography. J Am Coll Cardiol 2005;46:552–7.
8. Laudon DA, Vukov LF, Breen JF, et al. Use of electron-beam computed tomography in the evaluation of chest pain patients in the emergency department. Ann Emerg Med 1999;33:15–21.
9. Achenbach S, Daniel WG. Noninvasive coronary angiography-an acceptable alternative? N Engl J Med 2001;345:1909–10.
10. Giesler T, Baum U, Ropers D, et al. Noninvasive visualization of coronary arteries using contrast-enhanced multidetector CT: influence of heart rate on image quality and stenosis detection. AJR Am J Roentgenol 2002;179:911–6.
11. Stein PD, Beemath A, Kayali F, et al. Multidetector computed tomography for the diagnosis of coronary artery disease: a systematic review. Am J Med 2006;119:203–16.
12. Kopp AF, Schroeder S, Kuettner A, et al. Non-invasive coronary angiography with high resolution multidetector-row computed tomography. Eur Heart J 2002;23:1714–25.
13. Budoff M, Achenbach S, Blumenthal R, et al. Assessment of coronary artery disease by cardiac computed tomography: a scientific statement from the American Heart Association Committee on Cardiovascular Imaging and Intervention, Council on Cardiovascular Radiology and Intervention, and Committee on Cardiac Imaging, Council on Clinical Cardiology. Circulation 2006;114:1761–91.
14. Kuettner A, Beck T, Drosch T, et al. Diagnostic accuracy of noninvasive coronary imaging using 16-detector slice spiral computed tomography with 188 ms temporal resolution. J Am Coll Cardiol 2005;45:123–7.
15. Dewey M, Laule M, Krug L, et al. Multisegment and halfscan reconstruction of 16-slice computed tomography for detection of coronary artery stenoses. Invest Radiol 2004;39:223–9.
16. Kuettner A, Trabold T, Schroeder S, et al. Noninvasive detection of coronary lesions using 16-detector multislice spiral computed tomography technology: initial clinical results. J Am Coll Cardiol 2004;44:1230–7.
17. Mollet NR, Cademartiri F, Krestin GP, et al. Improved diagnostic accuracy with 16-row multi-slice computed tomography coronary angiography. J Am Coll Cardiol 2005;45:128–32.
18. Mollet NR, Cademartiri F, Nieman K, et al. Multislice spiral computed tomography coronary angiography in patients with stable angina pectoris. J Am Coll Cardiol 2004;43:2265–70.
19. Martuscelli E, Romagnoli A, D'Eliseo A, et al. Accuracy of thin-slice computed tomography in the detection of coronary stenoses. Eur Heart J 2004;25:1043–8.
20. Leschka S, Alkadhi H, Plass A, et al. Accuracy of MSCT coronary angiography with 64-slice technology: first experience. Eur Heart J 2005;26:1482–7.
21. Leber AW, Knez A, von Ziegler F, et al. Quantification of obstructive and nonobstructive coronary lesions by 64-slice computed tomography: a comparative study with quantitative coronary angiography and intravascular ultrasound. J Am Coll Cardiol 2005;46:147–54.
22. Mollet NR, Cademartiri F, van Mieghem CA, et al. High-resolution spiral computed tomography coronary angiography in patients referred for diagnostic conventional coronary angiography. Circulation 2005;112:2318–23.
23. Pugliese F, Mollet NR, Runza G, et al. Diagnostic accuracy of non-invasive 64-slice CT coronary angiography in patients with stable angina pectoris. Eur Radiol 2006;16:575–82.
24. Ropers D, Rixe J, Anders K, et al. Usefulness of multidetector row spiral computed tomography with 64- × 0.6-mm collimation and 330-ms rotation

for the noninvasive detection of significant coronary artery stenoses. Am J Cardiol 2006;97:343–8.

25. White CS, Kuo D. Chest pain in the emergency department: role of multidetector CT. Radiology 2007;245:672–81.

26. Stein PD, Fowler SE, Goodman LR, et al. Multidetector computed tomography for acute pulmonary embolism. N Engl J Med 2006;354:2317–27.

27. Nienaber CA, Eagle KA. Aortic dissection: new frontiers in diagnosis and management. I. From etiology to diagnostic strategies. Circulation 2003;108:628–35.

28. Agatston A, Janowitz WR, Hildner FJ, et al. Quantification of coronary artery calcium using ultrafast computed tomography. J Am Coll Cardiol 1990;15: 827–32.

29. Rumberger JA, Brundage BH, Rader DJ, et al. Electron beam computed tomographic coronary calcium scanning: a review and guidelines for use in asymptomatic persons. Mayo Clin Proc 1999;74:243–52.

30. Detrano R, Guerci AD, Carr JJ, et al. Coronary calcium as a predictor of coronary events in four racial or ethnic groups. N Engl J Med 2008;358: 1336–45.

31. McLaughlin VV, Balogh T, Rich S. Utility of electron beam computed tomography to stratify patients presenting to the emergency room with chest pain. Am J Cardiol 1999;84:327–8.

32. Georgiou D, Budoff MJ, Kaufer E, et al. Screening patients with chest pain in the emergency department using electron beam tomography: a follow-up study. J Am Coll Cardiol 2001;38:105–10.

33. Greenland P, Bonow RO, Brundage BH, et al. ACCF/AHA 2007 clinical expert consensus document on coronary artery calcium scoring by computed tomography in global cardiovascular risk assessment and in evaluation of patients with chest pain. J Am Coll Cardiol 2007;49:378–402.

34. White HD, Norris RM, Brown MA, et al. Left ventricular end-systolic volume as the major determinant of survival after recovery from myocardial infarction. Circulation 1987;76:44–51.

35. Hammermeister KE, DeRouen TA, Dodge HT. Variables predictive of survival in patients with coronary disease: selection by univariate and multivariate analyses from the clinical, electrocardiographic, exercise, arteriographic, and quantitative angiographic evaluations. Circulation 1979;59:421–30.

36. Halliburton S, Petersilka M, Schvartzman P, et al. Validation of left ventricular volume and ejection fraction measurement with multi-slice computed tomography: comparison to cine magnetic resonance imaging. Radiology 2001;221(P):452.

37. Treede H, Becker C, Reichenspurner H, et al. Multidetector computed tomography (MDCT) in coronary surgery: first experience with a new tool for diagnosis of coronary artery disease. Ann Thorac Surg 2002;74:S1398–402.

38. Burgstahler C, Keuttner A, Kopp AF, et al. Non-invasive evaluation of coronary artery bypass grafts using multi-slice computed tomography: initial experience. Int J Cardiol 2003;90:275–80.

39. Nieman K, Pattynama PM, Rensing BJ, et al. Evaluation of patients after coronary artery bypass surgery: CT angiographic assessment of grafts and coronary arteries. Radiology 2003;229:749–56.

40. Flohr T, Stierstorfer K, Raupach R, et al. Performance evaluation of a 64-slice CT system with z-flying focal spot. Rofo 2004;176:1803–10.

41. Miller J, Rochitte C, Dewey M, et al. Diagnostic performance of coronary angiography by 64-row CT. N Engl J Med 2008;359:2324–36.

42. Onuma Y, Tanabe K, Chihara R, et al. Evaluation of coronary artery bypass grafts and native coronary arteries using 64-slice multidetector computed tomography. Am Heart J 2007;154:519–26.

43. Meyer TS, Martinoff S, Hadamitzky M, et al. Improved noninvasive assessment of coronary artery bypass grafts with 64-slice computed tomographic angiography in an unselected patient population. J Am Coll Cardiol 2007;49:946–50.

44. Malagutti P, Nieman K, Meijboom WB, et al. Use of 64-slice CT in symptomatic patients after coronary bypass surgery: evaluation of grafts and coronary arteries. Eur Heart J 2007;28:1879–85.

45. Ma E, Yang Z, Wang Q, et al. Clinical application of 64-slice CT in evaluation of vessel before and after coronary artery bypass graft surgery. Sheng Wu Yi Xue Gong Cheng Xue Za Zhi 2009;26:491–5 [in Chinese].

46. Liu ZY, Gao CQ, Li BJ, et al. Diagnostic study on the coronary artery bypass grafts lesions using 64 multi-slice computed tomography angiography. Zhonghua Wai Ke Za Zhi 2008;15(46):245–7 [in Chinese].

47. Pugliese F, Cademartiri F, van Mieghem C, et al. Multidetector CT for visualization of coronary stents. Radiographics 2006;26:887–904.

48. Nieman K, Cademartiri F, Raaijmakers R, et al. Noninvasive angiographic evaluation of coronary stents with multi-slice spiral computed tomography. Herz 2003;28:136–42.

49. Gerber BL, Belge B, Legros GJ, et al. Characterization of acute and chronic myocardial infarcts by multidetector computed tomography. Comparison with contrast-enhanced magnetic resonance. Circulation 2006;113:823–33.

50. Mahnken AH, Koos R, Katoh M, et al. Assessment of myocardial viability in reperfused acute myocardial infarction using 16-slice computed tomography in comparison to magnetic resonance imaging. J Am Coll Cardiol 2005;45:2042–7.

51. Habis M, Capderou A, Ghostine S, et al. Acute myocardial infarction early viability assessment by 64-slice computed tomography immediately after coronary angiography: comparison with low-dose

dobutamine echocardiography. J Am Coll Cardiol 2007;49:1178–85.

52. Cronin P, Sneider M, Kazerooni E, et al. MDCT of the left atrium and pulmonary veins in planning radiofrequency ablation for atrial fibrillation: a how-to guide. AJR Am J Roentgenol 2004; 183:767–78.

53. Hocini M, Sanders P, Jais P, et al. Techniques for curative treatment of atrial fibrillation. J Cardiovasc Electrophysiol 2004;15:1467–71.

54. Sundaram B, Patel S, Bogot N, et al. Anatomy and terminology for the interpretation and reporting of cardiac MDCT: part 1, structured report, coronary calcium screening, and coronary artery anatomy. AJR Am J Roentgenol 2009;192:574–83.

55. Hendel RC, Patel MR, Kramer CM, et al. ACCF/ACR/SCCT/SCMR/ASNC/NASCI/SCAI/SIR 2006 appropriateness criteria for cardiac computed tomography and cardiac magnetic resonance imaging: a report of the American College of Cardiology Foundation Quality Strategic Directions Committee Appropriateness Criteria Working Group, American College of Radiology, Society of Cardiovascular Computed Tomography, Society for Cardiovascular Magnetic Resonance, American Society of Nuclear Cardiology, North American Society for Cardiac Imaging, Society for Cardiovascular Angiography and Interventions, and Society of Interventional Radiology. J Am Coll Cardiol 2006;48:1475–97.

56. Angelini P, Velasco JA, Flamm S. Coronary anomalies: incidence, pathophysiology, and clinical relevance. Circulation 2002;105:2449–54.

57. Pelliccia A. Congenital coronary artery anomalies in young patients: new perspectives for timely identification. J Am Coll Cardiol 2001;37:598–600.

Cardiac Magnetic Resonance Imaging in Ischemic Heart Disease

Abigail May Khan, MD[a], Harold Litt, MD, PhD[a,b],
Victor Ferrari, MD[a], Yuchi Han, MD, MMSc[a,*]

KEYWORDS

- MR imaging • Ischemic heart disease
- Coronary artery disease • Acute ischemia
- Chronic ischemia

Coronary artery disease (CAD) is the leading cause of death in the adult population in the United States.[1] Whereas many patients with CAD are asymptomatic, some patients develop myocardial ischemia manifesting as angina, myocardial infarction (MI), or heart failure.[1] The identification of both symptomatic and asymptomatic individuals with CAD is of the utmost importance to clinicians, because there are now multiple therapies that can improve symptoms and reduce the risk of cardiovascular events and mortality in these patients.[2]

Imaging is an essential component of the management of suspected CAD, providing both diagnostic and prognostic information.[3,4] Whereas imaging modalities such as echocardiography, single-photon emission computed tomography (SPECT), and coronary angiography have been the mainstay of evaluation for patients for CAD for decades, cardiac magnetic resonance (CMR) imaging has recently emerged as a robust alternative.[5] CMR imaging is a versatile technique that uses a combination of radiofrequency pulses and magnetic field gradients to emphasize different structural and physiologic properties of tissue and can identify pathologic changes of disease processes such as edema and fibrosis.

A large body of preclinical and clinical evidence over the past 3 decades now supports the use of CMR imaging in the diagnosis and management of cardiac ischemia.[6] CMR imaging offers distinct benefits over other cardiac imaging modalities, including a lack of radiation exposure,[7,8] superior spatial resolution,[9] excellent reproducibility, and the ability to provide both anatomic and functional data in a single study.

In this review, we provide an overview of the data supporting the use of CMR imaging in the evaluation of ischemia in both acute and chronic settings, including recent developments in the field and important directions for future research. Detailed CMR imaging techniques and protocols have been reviewed elsewhere,[10,11] and are beyond the scope of this article.

INTRODUCTION TO CMR IMAGING SPECIFIC TECHNIQUES
Myocardial Edema

The brightness of the voxel of an acquired CMR image is directly proportional to the amount of signal measured in the receiver coils. Different MR sequences can be used to emphasize different tissue properties such as proton density, T1 relaxation time, and T2 relaxation time.[12] Normal tissues have relatively short T1 and T2 times, whereas fluids, such as blood or edema, have

The authors have nothing to disclose.

[a] Cardiovascular Division, Department of Medicine, University of Pennsylvania, 3400 Spruce Street, Philadelphia, PA 19103, USA
[b] Department of Radiology, University of Pennsylvania, 3400 Spruce Street, Philadelphia, PA 19103, USA
* Corresponding author.
E-mail address: yuchi.han@uphs.upenn.edu

PET Clin 6 (2011) 453–473
doi:10.1016/j.cpet.2011.10.002

relatively long T1 and T2 times.[12] A T2-weighted image sequence highlights myocardial edema as increased signal intensity in the myocardium.

Contrast-Enhanced CMR Imaging

Perfusion

CMR imaging can assess myocardial perfusion and stress-induced wall motion abnormalities, and therefore is an important tool for the diagnosis of stable CAD. Because of its short half-life and favorable safety profile, adenosine, a direct coronary vasodilator, is the most commonly used hyperemic agent in CMR perfusion imaging. In adenosine stress imaging, first pass of contrast through the left ventricular (LV) myocardium is obtained at rest and again at maximal hyperemia in the short and long axis planes, allowing for detection of areas with reduced perfusion.[13]

Late gadolinium enhancement

Late gadolinium enhancement (LGE) is a powerful technique to visualize myocardial necrosis with high resolution (**Fig. 1**).[9,14] In the acute setting, damage to cellular membranes results in the rapid distribution of gadolinium within the intracellular space, causing increased gadolinium enhancement in necrotic, as opposed to viable, myocardium.[15] In the chronic setting, expansion of the interstitial space occurs, and fibrosis or scarring replaces necrotic tissue, leading to increased gadolinium concentration in scar tissue.[16] This phenomenon, referred to as LGE, shows temporal stability, and can be used to quantify the extent of myocardial necrosis with a low intraobserver and

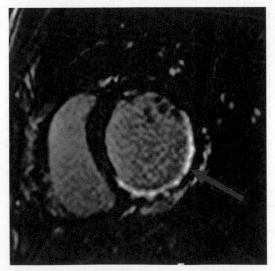

Fig. 1. CMR images in the short axis plane of a patient with inferolateral MI. *Arrow* points to the subendocardial LGE.

interobserver variability.[17] In a small study by Ricciardi and colleagues,[14] LGE detected discrete areas of myocardial necrosis with a mass as small as 0.7 g.

CMR IMAGING AND MI

Diagnosis of Acute MI

An estimated 900,000 MIs occur in the United States a year.[1] Individuals with acute MI, and especially subgroups such as diabetics, are at high risk for both early and late complications; therefore prompt diagnosis is of paramount importance.[18,19] The rapid diagnosis of acute coronary syndromes (ACS) is complicated by the fact that most patients presenting to the emergency department (ED) with chest pain do not have ACS, and the high prevalence of other syndromes that mimic MI.[20] Although clinical and laboratory assessment and the electrocardiogram (ECG) remain the cornerstone of ACS diagnosis, imaging is frequently indicated to increase diagnostic accuracy and facilitate therapy in many patients.[18,19,21]

Several studies have examined the use of CMR imaging in the detection of acute MI in the ED.[22,23] Kwong and colleagues[22] studied 161 low-risk individuals presenting with chest pain and suspected myocardial ischemia, performing CMR imaging within 12 hours of presentation. The presence of a wall motion abnormality (**Fig. 2**) or abnormal LGE had a sensitivity of 84% and a specificity of 85% for the diagnosis of MI, comparing favorably with the combination of ECG, TIMI (thrombolysis in myocardial infarction) risk score, and cardiac troponin. Cury and colleagues[23] performed CMR imaging with T2-weighted imaging to assess myocardial edema (**Fig. 3**) as an indicator for acute myocardial injury in 62 patients presenting to the ED with acute onset of chest pain and negative ECG and cardiac biomarkers, finding that CMR imaging provided additive value over clinical assessment and cardiovascular risk factors in this population. The mean duration of CMR imaging in this study was 32 ± 8 minutes, suggesting that the examination can be performed rapidly in the acute setting.[23] Perhaps equally as important, CMR imaging can also identify other causes of chest pain that may mimic acute MI, such as aortic dissection (**Fig. 4**),[24] myopericarditis (**Fig. 5**),[25] and stress (Takotsubo) cardiomyopathy (**Fig. 6**).[26]

Although acute ST elevation MI (STEMI) is an indication for emergent revascularization,[18] an early invasive strategy has not been shown to benefit all patients with unstable angina and non-STEMI (NSTEMI). An early invasive strategy is recommended for high-risk individuals, as defined by clinical risk tools such as the GRACE (Global

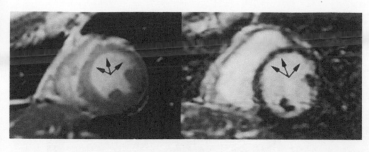

Fig. 2. CMR images of a patient with unstable angina and a 95% stenosis of the left anterior descending coronary artery. Akinetic anterior and anteroseptal walls appeared thinner at end-systole than other segments (*left*) with no LGE (*right*) (*arrows*). This situation indicates ischemic but not infarcted myocardium. (*Reprinted from* Kwong RY, Schussheim AE, Rekhraj S, et al. Detecting acute coronary syndrome in the emergency department with cardiac magnetic resonance imaging. Circulation 2003;107(4):533; with permission.)

Registry of Acute Coronary Events) score.[27] However, there are limitations to the use of a clinical risk score. To this end, Raman and colleagues[28] performed CMR imaging with T2-weighted edema imaging and LGE in 100 patients with non-ST elevation ACS- (NSTEMI and unstable angina) before percutaneous coronary intervention (PCI). The presence of myocardial edema in this study

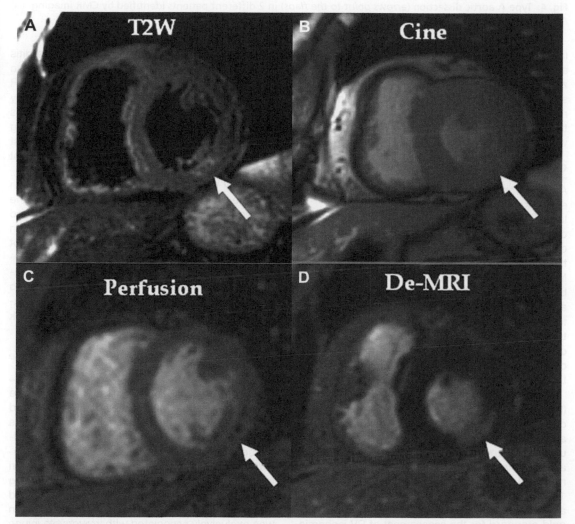

Fig. 3. Tissue characterization using CMR imaging in a patient with a non-ST elevation MI. A small area of T2 hyperintensity (*A*) in the inferolateral wall (myocardial edema) with associated subtle hypokinesis (*B*), a resting perfusion defect (*C*), and delayed hyperenhancement (*D*) in the same area (*arrows*). (*Reprinted from* Cury RC, Shash K, Nagurney JT, et al. Cardiac magnetic resonance with T2-weighted imaging improves detection of patients with acute coronary syndrome in the emergency department. Circulation 2008;118(8):841; with permission.)

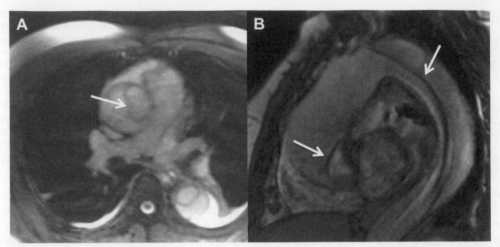

Fig. 4. Type A aortic dissection (*arrows point to the flaps*) in 2 different patients identified by CMR imaging. (*A*) An axial image. (*B*) A sagittal image.

(a marker of ischemia/reperfusion in that coronary artery territory) predicted the need for revascularization, whereas clinical markers, such as TIMI risk score and ECG changes, did not. This finding, if reproduced in the general population, has important implications for the management of patients with NSTEMI.

Characterization of MI and its Sequelae

Another important use of CMR imaging is in differentiating acute from chronic MI (**Fig. 7**).[29–31] A large, multicenter trial of patients by Kim and colleagues[29] reported a sensitivity of 99% for the detection of acute MI (defined as ≤16 days after the event) and 94% for the detection of chronic MI (>16 days after the event). Infarct localization by CMR imaging compares favorably with coronary angiography, which is the current gold standard for detection of coronary stenoses.[30,32] In addition to infarct location, CMR imaging can accurately determine infarct size and differentiate subendocardial from transmural infarction (**Fig. 8**), information that cannot be obtained by angiography.[29]

The presence of right ventricular (RV) infarction (**Fig. 9**) is associated with an increased risk of cardiogenic shock, arrhythmias, and mortality in acute MI.[33] Imaging of the thin-walled and uniquely shaped RV is difficult with most currently available imaging modalities, and RV infarction may not be reliably detected on conventional 12-lead electrocardiography. CMR imaging allows a major advance for RV imaging, and is now the gold standard for the assessment of RV ischemia and function.[34]

CMR imaging can accurately detect many sequelae of acute MI, including intraventricular thrombus (**Fig. 10**),[35,36] papillary muscle infarction

(**Fig. 11**),[37] pericardial effusion,[36] and pericarditis (see **Fig. 10**).[36] When compared with transthoracic and transesophageal echocardiography, CMR imaging has a higher sensitivity and specificity for detection of LV thrombus,[38] and therefore is the test of choice for this diagnosis. CMR imaging can be safely performed at 1.5 T (the most commonly used field strength) within days of stent implantation.[39]

Several recent studies have led to recognition that the incidence of silent MIs, defined as the presence of myocardial scar without a recognized episode of chest pain, is relatively high in population-based studies,[40,41] although it is not clear that myocardial scar is related to atherosclerosis in all individuals.[42] The presence of unrecognized MI adds incremental prognostic value to traditional measures,[43,44] and identifies a population that should be targeted for aggressive risk modification.

Characterization of Reversible and Irreversible Injury

CMR imaging can identify myocardial hemorrhage (**Fig. 12**) after acute MI, a finding that is associated with irreversible vascular injury and predicts adverse LV remodeling.[45–48] In a proof-of-concept study, Rehwald and colleagues[16] examined changes in gadolinium concentration in infarcted and at-risk areas of myocardium using electron probe radiograph microanalysis and found that increased gadolinium concentration was exclusively associated with irreversible injury. LGE can distinguish irreversible from reversible myocardial damage soon after MI,[15,16,49] assisting in identification of both high-risk and low-risk individuals after MI.

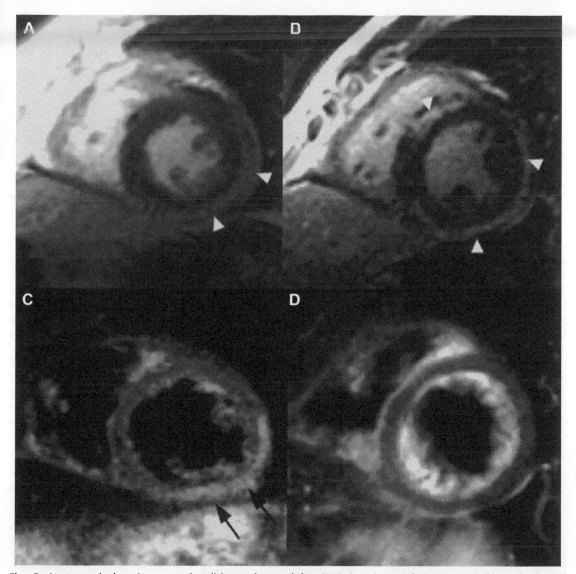

Fig. 5. Acute and chronic myopericarditis as detected by CMR imaging techniques. LGE (*A* and *B*) and T2-weighted images (*C* and *D*) were obtained in 2 patients. The first patient (*A* and *C*) has no epicardial LGE and high myocardial signal intensity on T2-weighted imaging in the corresponding area, indicating acute myocarditis (*arrowheads* in *A*, and *arrows* in *C*). Second patient (*B* and *D*) had epicardial LGE in 2 different regions (anteroseptal and anterolateral extending to inferior) with no increased signal intensity on T2-weighted imaging indicating chronic myocarditis (*arrowheads* in *C*). (*Modified from* Abdel-Aty H, Boye P, Zagrosek A, et al. Diagnostic performance of cardiovascular magnetic resonance in patients with suspected acute myocarditis: comparison of different approaches. J Am Coll Cardiol 2005;45(11):1820; with permission.)

Despite successful recanalization of the culprit artery with percutaneous coronary intervention, a significant minority of individuals do not have complete reperfusion of the infarcted territory. This phenomenon, called no reflow, is believed to be related to microvascular obstruction (MVO) and has been correlated with adverse outcomes.[50] MVO (see **Fig. 12**) can be detected by CMR imaging shortly after MI.[51–53] When compared with angiographic and ECG correlates of reperfusion, measurement of MVO on CMR imaging is a stronger predictor of functional recovery.[52] Furthermore, the presence of MVO may be a better predictor of prognosis based on myocardial recovery, cardiovascular complications, and mortality than infarct size and LV ejection fraction (LVEF).[51–53]

The most powerful indicator of the efficacy of reperfusion therapy is the myocardial salvage

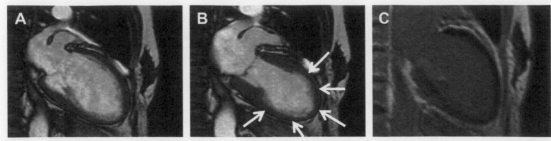

Fig. 6. CMR imaging of Takotsubo stress cardiomyopathy. (*A*) 2 chamber view of the heart in diastole. (*B*) 2 chamber view of the heart in systole. *Arrows* point to the area of severe hypokinesis (*apical ballooning*). (*C*) Late gadolinium enhancement imaging demonstrated no enhancement in the area of apical ballooning. (*Modified from* Eitel I, Behrendt F, Schindler K, et al. Differential diagnosis of suspected apical ballooning syndrome using contrast-enhanced magnetic resonance imaging. Eur Heart J 2008;29(21):2655; with permission.)

index (MSI), which is a measure of the final infarct size compared with the amount of at-risk myocardium. This measure, traditionally obtained by SPECT, is of prognostic significance and has been an important outcome measure in clinical trials.[54] However, SPECT measurement of MSI in the peri-infarct period is often not feasible.[55] In a recent paper, Eitel and colleagues[55] assessed the MSI in 208 patients after PCI for STEMI using T2-weighted CMR imaging and LGE obtained within 1 to 4 days after MI. The investigators found that the MSI, obtained by CMR imaging using (myocardial edema volume − LGE volume)/myocardial edema volume was a powerful predictor of major adverse cardiovascular events (MACE), defined as a composite of death, reinfarction, and new heart failure over 6 months of follow-up.

Because of its superior spatial resolution, CMR imaging can reliably detect both transmural and subendocardial infarcts.[9] In a study by Beek and colleagues,[56] 30 patients underwent CMR imaging after acute reperfused MI. The likelihood of recovery of function of segments without LGE was 50 times higher than for those with greater than 75% LGE, a finding supported by other studies.[15,57] Transmural infarction has also been shown to be negatively associated with recovery of contractile function.[58]

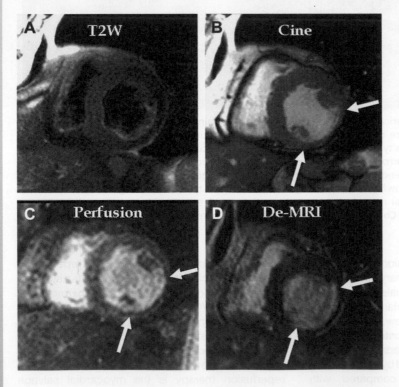

Fig. 7. Chronic MI in a patient with previous left circumflex territory MI and no ACS. CMR imaging showed an absence of high signal intensity on T2-weighted imaging (*A*), an area of LV thinning on cine imaging (*B*), perfusion defect (*C*), and subendocardial delayed hyperenhancement (*D*) in the inferolateral and inferior walls consistent with a chronic myocardial infarct (*arrows*). (*Reprinted from* Cury RC, Shash K, Nagurney JT, et al. Cardiac magnetic resonance with T2-weighted imaging improves detection of patients with acute coronary syndrome in the emergency department. Circulation 2008;118(8):842; with permission.)

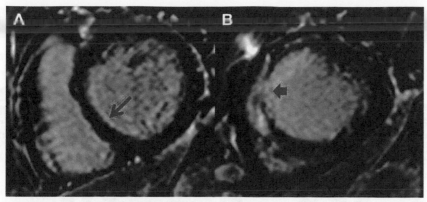

Fig. 8. In a patient who presented with acute MI, both subendocardial basal inferoseptal (*A, long arrow*) and transmural infarction (apical septal) (*B, short arrow*) are found on LGE imaging.

MI results in important changes in LV geometry, a process referred to as adverse remodeling. Remodeling is associated with poor outcomes, and prevention of adverse remodeling is a target of many post-MI therapies.[59] CMR imaging measures, such as the MSI or the presence of MVO, may serve as surrogate end points for clinical trials, or identify individuals at high risk for adverse remodeling who may benefit from aggressive therapies.[60–62]

Comparison with Other Modalities

Although the results of small studies are promising, several technical and logistical issues limit the wider implementation of CMR imaging

for diagnosis of acute myocardial ischemia. The performance and interpretation of CMR imaging requires specialized training, and access remains limited in the ED.[63] Furthermore, cardiac computed tomography (CT) can be performed more rapidly and can also identify other potentially life-threatening causes of chest pain, such as aortic dissection and pulmonary embolism, although it entails the risk of ionizing radiation exposure and iodinated contrast agents.[64] CMR imaging is unlikely to surpass CT imaging as the primary myocardial imaging modality in the emergency setting. However, CMR imaging likely has an important role in the care of selected patients.

With regard to the detection of MI and myocardial scar, CMR imaging has been compared with both SPECT and positron emission tomography

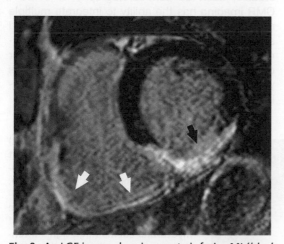

Fig. 9. An LGE image showing acute inferior MI (*black arrow*) with RV involvement (*white arrows*) shows hyperenhancement (no viability) in these areas. (*Reprinted from* Hombach V, Grebe O, Merkle N, et al. Sequelae of acute myocardial infarction regarding cardiac structure and function and their prognostic significance as assessed by magnetic resonance imaging. Eur Heart J 2005;26(6):522; with permission.)

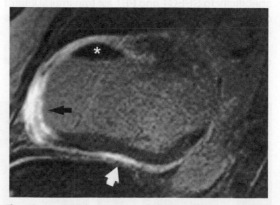

Fig. 10. An LGE image in a patient with a large anterior MI (*black arrow*). Both LV thrombus (*asterisk*) and pericarditis (*white arrow*) are sequelae of the MI that are present in this patient. (*Reprinted from* Hombach V, Grebe O, Merkle N, et al. Sequelae of acute myocardial infarction regarding cardiac structure and function and their prognostic significance as assessed by magnetic resonance imaging. Eur Heart J 2005; 26(6):552; with permission.)

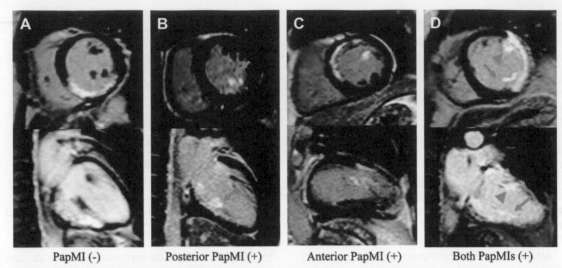

PapMI (-)   Posterior PapMI (+)   Anterior PapMI (+)   Both PapMIs (+)

Fig. 11. LGE CMR images from patients with STEMI involving RCA (*A, B*), LAD (*C*), and left circumflex (*D*). No papillary muscle infarction is shown in patient A. Posterior papillary muscle infarction (*B*), anterior papillary muscle infarction (*C*), and bilateral papillary muscle infarction (*D*) (*arrow*, posterior papillary muscle; *arrowhead*, anterior papillary muscle). (*Reprinted from* Tanimoto T, Imanishi T, Kitabata H, et al. Prevalence and clinical significance of papillary muscle infarction detected by late gadolinium-enhanced magnetic resonance imaging in patients with ST-segment elevation myocardial infarction. Circulation 2010;122(22):2283; with permission.)

(PET) imaging prospectively with promising results. In a study of 31 patients with known ischemic cardiomyopathy, MR detection of myocardial scar was correlated with scar detection by PET imaging.[65] The ability of CMR imaging to detect transmural infarction is also equivalent to SPECT imaging, which is still the modality most widely used in cardiology practice.[9] Although CMR imaging shows equivalent sensitivity and specificity to SPECT and PET for transmural infarct detection, it also offers distinct diagnostic benefits over these modalities.

CMR imaging measures that correlated with outcome after MI include the presence of hemorrhagic myocardium and MVO, and the degree of myocardial salvage.[45,51,53,66] CMR imaging also provides information about more traditional markers of risk, such as infarct size and LVEF.[67] Although these measures have historically been obtained with other imaging studies, such as echocardiography or SPECT, CMR imaging has the ability to integrate multiple risk markers with greater reproducibility and spatial resolution than these conventional techniques, and therefore may be a better predictor of long-term outcome. However, this theory has yet to be assessed prospectively by a large clinical trial.

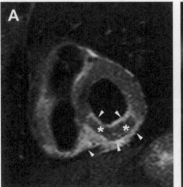

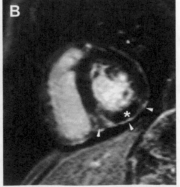

Fig. 12. Short-axis T2-weighted (*A*) and LGE (*B*) images from a patient with acute inferior MI with myocardial hemorrhage and MVO. Myocardial hemorrhage is represented by the central hypointense area (*A, asterisks*) within the area of myocardial edema (high signal intensity) that extends into the right ventricle (*A, arrowheads*). A large area of transmural necrosis (*B, arrowheads*) with a large core of MVO (*asterisk*) is shown on the LGE image. (*Reprinted from* Ganame J, Messalli G, Dymarkowski S, et al. Impact of myocardial haemorrhage on left ventricular function and remodelling in patients with reperfused acute myocardial infarction. Eur Heart J 2009;30(12):1443; with permission.)

ASSESSMENT OF MYOCARDIAL ISCHEMIA IN STABLE CAD
CMR Perfusion Imaging

The diagnostic performance of CMR perfusion imaging has been directly compared with coronary angiography,[5,68–72] SPECT,[70,72,73] (**Table 1**), and PET imaging.[5] MR-IMPACT (Magnetic Resonance Imaging for Myocardial Perfusion Assessment in Coronary Artery Disease Trial),[72] a trial performed at 33 European centers, is the largest study of CMR perfusion to date. In this study, 234 patients underwent CMR perfusion, SPECT, and coronary angiography. The diagnostic performance of CMR imaging was good, with an area under the receiver operating characteristic curve of 0.86.[72] In the entire population of participants, CMR imaging performed better than SPECT for single-vessel and multivessel disease (**Fig. 13**). Most recently, Lockie and colleagues[74] compared 3-T stress perfusion CMR imaging with fractional flow reserve (FFR) in the assessment of myocardial perfusion and found a sensitivity of 0.80 and a specificity of 0.89 for the detection of hemodynamically significant coronary stenoses.

The prognostic value of CMR perfusion has been examined in several studies.[4,75,76] Bodi and colleagues reported that abnormal stress perfusion at CMR imaging in response to dipyridamole was associated with MACE in more than 400 patients with known or suspected CAD.[4,75] These findings have been reproduced using adenosine stress perfusion in more than 500 patients,[4] and in an even larger cohort by Krittayaphong and colleagues.[76]

A meta-analysis examined the diagnostic performance of both stress perfusion MR and imaging of stress-induced wall motion abnormalities, including 37 studies with a combined total of more than 2000 patients. In this analysis, stress perfusion had a sensitivity of 0.83 and a specificity of 0.86 for the detection of ischemia in a population with a relatively high prevalence of CAD. These numbers are comparable with, if not superior to, other stress imaging modalities.[70,73,77] Patients with normal adenosine stress perfusion CMR imaging had no diagnosis of CAD or adverse outcome at 1-year follow-up in individuals who presented with chest pain to the ED.[78] Therefore, a negative stress perfusion study obviates further testing in most patients.

Although it is well understood that not all patients benefit from revascularization for stable CAD, the identification of individuals who derive the greatest therapeutic benefit is an ongoing challenge. MR-INFORM (MR Perfusion Imaging to Guide Management of Patients With Stable Coronary Artery Disease) is an ongoing trial comparing MR perfusion and FFR-based management in patients with stable CAD. The primary end point of the trial is the occurrence of MACE at 1-year follow-up.

Dobutamine Stress Magnetic Resonance

Dobutamine stress testing, which can be performed with echocardiography, SPECT, or CMR imaging, is a test in which a graded dose of dobutamine is administered per a standard protocol during imaging. Ischemia is detected when wall motion abnormalities develop under stress. Although dobutamine stress echocardiography (DSE) has been well validated, CMR imaging offers better spatial resolution and is less subject to limitations posed by patient body habitus. In a single-center study in which dobutamine stress magnetic resonance (DSMR), DSE, and coronary angiography were successfully performed in most

---

Table 1
Comparison of selected studies on first-pass stress perfusion CMR imaging and SPECT imaging for the detection of coronary artery stenoses using coronary angiography as the gold standard

Author, Year	Study Design	N	Stress Modality	AUC CMR	AUC SPECT
Ishida et al,[70] 2003	Single-center, 99mTc TF or MIBI or 201Tl SPECT	69	Dipyridamole	0.91	0.75
Sakuma et al,[73] 2005	Single-center, individuals with suspected CAD, 201Tl SPECT	40	Dipyridamole	0.86	0.79
Schwitter et al,[72] 2008	Multicenter, randomized, double-blind, 99mTc or 201Tl SPECT	234	Adenosine	0.86	0.75

Abbreviations: AUC, area under the receiver operating characteristic curve; MIBI, methoxyisobutylisonitrile; Tc, technetium; TF, tesoformin; Tl, thallium.

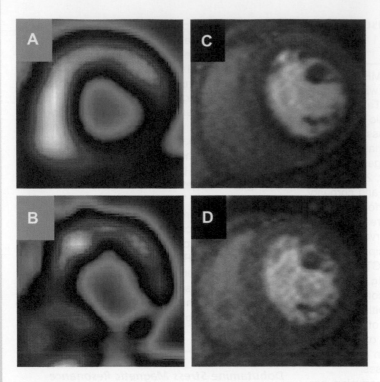

Fig. 13. Perfusion CMR imaging and SPECT imaging in a patient who had multivessel disease. The SPECT (*Left,* *A,* Stress image; *B,* rest image) showed the fixed inferior and inferolateral defect. The CMR imaging stress perfusion image (*C*) showed perfusion defects in the inferoseptal, inferior and inferolateral territories, and rest perfusion (*D*) showed fixed defect in the inferior territory. SPECT imaging missed reversible inferoseptal and inferolateral defects in this patient, who went on to CABG based on CMR imaging with improved LVEF after revascularization.

patients with suspected CAD, DSMR yielded a higher diagnostic accuracy than DSE.[79] This result has been reproduced by multiple other groups.[80–84] These studies support the use of DSMR in individuals with limited echocardiographic windows, a population that would previously have required imaging with PET or SPECT.[82]

As with perfusion MR, abnormal DSMR is predictive of MACE, and a normal DSMR is strongly correlated with event-free survival.[4] DSMR is both feasible and safe in most patients.[85] The results of DSMR are reproducible,[86] and interobserver variability is low at experienced centers.[81,86] In 1 study directly comparing stress perfusion MR and DSMR, the tests performed similarly with respect to prediction of MACE.[4] Although the addition of stress perfusion imaging to a DSMR protocol improved sensitivity, it did not improve overall diagnostic accuracy and increased the false-positive rate.[87] Therefore, there does not seem to be an additional benefit of performing stress perfusion during DSMR.

In an attempt to determine the incremental prognostic value of multiple CMR imaging parameters for the detection of adverse cardiac events, Bingham and Hachamovitch[88] prospectively assessed 908 patients who were followed for a median of 2.6 years after CMR imaging with adenosine stress perfusion and LGE imaging in addition to functional imaging. This study confirmed that CMR

imaging results add prognostic value over pre-CMR imaging data and also showed that multiple CMR imaging parameters (assessment of stress perfusion, viability, cardiac flow, and LV structure and function) provided complementary, not overlapping, information.[88]

CMR Imaging Exercise Stress Testing

Exercise stress testing is preferred over stress perfusion and dobutamine stress testing because it provides information about functional status and increased prognostic value. Because of the technical constraints of MR-compatible equipment and logistics of imaging at the same location before and after exercise, access to CMR exercise stress testing has been limited. However, protocols have now been developed, and will likely be used with increased frequency in the future.[84,89]

MR Coronary Angiography

MR assessment of perfusion provides indirect evidence for the presence of coronary artery stenoses; however, evaluation of the patient with suspected CAD may require direct assessment of coronary anatomy. Although direct visualization of the coronary vasculature using cardiac catheterization is the current gold standard for the evaluation of CAD, the invasive nature of the procedure carries inherent risk to the patient. CT angiography is a well validated technique for the detection of stenoses, but does not provide the wealth of information about cardiac structure, function, and tissue characterization available with CMR imaging.[90]

Several investigators have examined the use of MR coronary angiography (MRCA) for detection of coronary stenoses.[74,91–93] In an early multicenter study, MRCA reliably detected CAD in the proximal and middle arterial segments compared with traditional angiography, suggesting that it can reliably exclude left main or triple vessel disease.[91] MRCA has several important technical limitations that preclude its wider use.[90,92] More recent research has focused on technological advances, such as improved respiratory gating techniques, higher field strength, and the use of contrast with higher relaxivity, to increase signal-to-noise ratio, and which may improve the accuracy, sensitivity, and feasibility of MRCA (**Fig. 14**).[92–95]

In addition to MRCA and stress perfusion, CMR imaging has been used to quantify myocardial blood flow in hibernating myocardium, although the clinical applications of this technique are in the early stages of development.[96] A thought-provoking study published recently by Kelle and colleagues[97] examined the use of 3-T CMR imaging to assess coronary artery distensibility in individuals with and without CAD. The investigators showed that it is possible to noninvasively quantify coronary artery distensibility and differentiate between normal and atherosclerotic vessels. The clinical relevance of this finding is intriguing, but has yet to be shown.

MYOCARDIAL VIABILITY

The presence of viable myocardium after MI predicts both outcome and response to revascularization.[98–101] Although a substudy from the recently

published STICH (Surgical Treatment for Ischemic Heart Failure) trial did not show a benefit to viability assessment with SPECT or dobutamine echocardiography before coronary artery bypass graft (CABG) surgery, viability testing is supported by American Heart Association guidelines and is still an integral component of the management of CAD.[102]

Myocardial viability is assessed using dobutamine echocardiography, SPECT, PET, or CMR imaging. Two major CMR imaging techniques are currently in use: LGE and low-dose dobutamine stress cine imaging. In a landmark study by Kim and colleagues,[103] LGE predicted the presence of reversible myocardial dysfunction before surgical or percutaneous revascularization. In a direct comparison of CMR imaging and SPECT, 20 patients with impaired LVEF before CABG were assessed.[104] The sensitivity of LGE for the recovery of contractile function 6 months after surgery was 99%, compared with 86% for SPECT.[104] In a related study, Kitagawa and colleagues[105] performed LGE and SPECT imaging in 22 patients after acute MI and found that the sensitivity, specificity, and accuracy of LGE was superior to SPECT. CMR imaging has subsequently been compared with [18F]-fluorodeoxyglucose (FDG)-PET (**Fig. 15**), which showed the equivalence of LGE and FDG-PET for prediction of myocardial functional improvement.[65,106–108] The direct comparison of CMR imaging with nuclear viability assessment is summarized in **Table 2**. In addition, LGE and FDG-PET may be additive to predict functional recovery after revascularization, which was examined in a study of 19 patients after MI.[109] In this study, both metabolic activity (as assessed by FDG-PET) and tissue composition (as assessed by LGE) helped discriminate classes of dysfunctional myocardium, in which metabolically active segments with a thick viable rim on LGE were most likely to recover function.[109] Further research in larger populations is

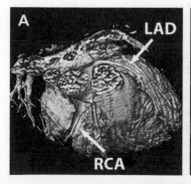
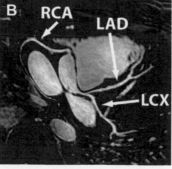

Fig. 14. Whole-heart contrast-enhanced coronary MR imaging. Three-dimensional volume-rendered (*A*) and reformatted (*B*) whole-heart steady-state free precession coronary artery images after a bolus injection of gadobenate dimeglumine in a healthy subject. All 3 major coronary arteries are clearly depicted. (*Reprinted from* Hu P, Chan J, Ngo LH, et al. Contrast-enhanced whole-heart coronary MRI with bolus infusion of gadobenate dimeglumine at 1.5 T. Magn Reson Med 2011;65(2): 397; with permission.)

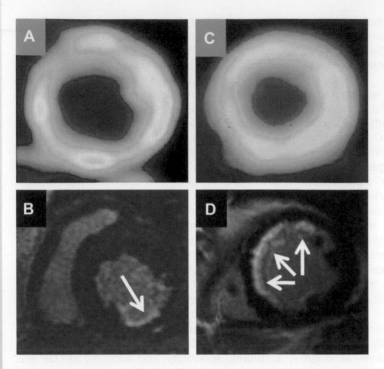

Fig. 15. PET and LGE CMR images in a patient with an inferolateral wall motion abnormality (*A* and *B*) and another patient with an anteroseptal wall motion abnormality (*C* and *D*). FDG-PET (*A* and *C*) on both patients were interpreted as normal myocardial viability, whereas LGE CMR showed subendocardial infarction (*arrows*). (*Courtesy of* Torsten Sommer, MD, German Red Cross Hospital, Neuwied, Germany.)

required to determine whether there is an incremental benefit of both FDG-PET and LGE assessment after MI in clinical practice.

Low-dose dobutamine stress cine imaging uses a dose of 5 to 10 mcg/kg/min of dobutamine to assess the contractile reserve of dysfunctional but viable myocardium, in contrast to high-dose dobutamine stress test (with doses up to 40 mcg/kg/min plus optional atropine), which is used to detect myocardial ischemia. A positive response in CMR imaging requires an identifiable increase in wall motion or thickening; this finding is as effective as low-dose dobutamine transesophageal echocardiography, but is less sensitive (although more specific) than nuclear techniques to predict functional recovery.[110,111]

Cardiac resynchronization therapy (CRT) improves outcomes in some, but not all, patients with severe LV dysfunction and heart failure.[112] The extent of myocardial viability as shown with low-dose dobutamine infusion[113] and the presence of scar tissue are related to the response to CRT.[114] A retrospective study reported that localization of LV lead tip and myocardial scar using LGE was associated with outcome, suggesting that perhaps CMR imaging could be used to guide lead placement.[115] Prospective studies are being performed to confirm this finding. In addition to scar location, coronary vein anatomy, which has significant individual variation, can be imaged

before lead implantation to guide lateral lead placement in CRT therapy, particularly in patients who do not have a suitable posterolateral vein; an epicardial approach may be favored rather an a percutaneous approach (**Fig. 16**).[116]

LIMITATIONS OF CMR IMAGING

CMR imaging continues to grow at a rapid pace. Improvements in MR technology have greatly expanded the diagnostic potential of CMR imaging, and numerous studies have now validated CMR imaging against other modalities and shown that it is a powerful predictor of prognosis and cardiac outcomes. However, several technological and logistical issues regarding the wider use of CMR imaging remain, including broader dissemination of education and expertise.

Imaging Protocols for the Rapid Diagnosis of Ischemia

The length of time required to obtain a CMR imaging study has limited the use of this technology, especially in acutely ill or unstable patients. However, rapid imaging protocols do exist.[117] The development of a protocol that uses state-of-the-art imaging techniques and scanners to rapidly identify acute MI without sacrificing diagnostic accuracy would be a significant advancement in the field.

Table 2
Comparison of selected studies on contrast-enhanced CMR imaging and PET/SPECT for the assessment of myocardial viability as defined by functional recovery

Author, Year	Study Population	N	Nuclear Study	Sensitivity, CMR (%)	Specificity, CMR (%)	PPV CMR (%)	NPV CMR (%)	Sensitivity, PET/SPECT (%)	Specificity, PET/SPECT (%)	PPV PET/SPECT (%)	NPV PET/SPECT (%)
Kitagawa et al,[105] 2003	Recent acute MI	22	^{201}Tl SPECT	98	75	92	93	90	54	85	66
Gutberlet et al,[104] 2005	Chronic ischemic heart disease	20	^{201}Tl SPECT	99	94	99	94	86	68	94	44
Kuhl et al,[107] 2006	Chronic ischemic heart disease	29	^{18}F-FDG PET/^{99m}Tc MIBI SPECT	97	68	73	93	87	76	73	77
Wu et al,[108] 2007	Chronic ischemic heart disease	41	^{18}F-FDG PET/^{201}Tl SPECT	92	45	72	79	60	99	77	97

Abbreviations: MIBI, methoxyisobutylisonitrile; NPV, negative predictive value; PPV, positive predictive value; Tc, technetium; Tl, thallium.

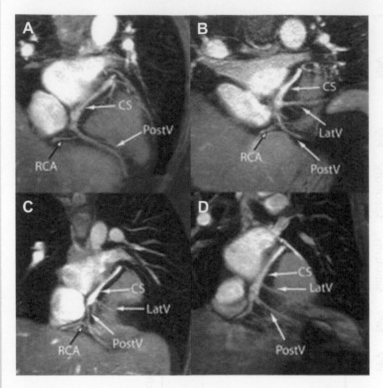

Fig. 16. Coronary vein imaging. The variations in the coronary venous anatomy in branching point, angle, and diameter of different tributaries of coronary sinus can be observed during the systolic rest period. Variation may have implications in transvenous versus epicardial approaches for left-sided lead implantation. For example, subject (*A*) has no visible lateral vein (LatV). CS, coronary sinus; PostV, posterior vein; RCA, right coronary artery. (*Reprinted from* Nezafat R, Han Y, Peters DC, et al. Coronary magnetic resonance vein imaging: imaging contrast, sequence, and timing. Magn Reson Med 2007; 58(6):1204; with permission.)

Validation of CMR Imaging Results in Multiple Populations

Few investigators have addressed the use of CMR imaging for ischemia detection outside clinical trial populations, which are predominantly male. A recent study by Gebker and colleagues[80] compared the diagnostic performance of DSMR in women with that in men and found that it was independent of gender. Although this finding is reassuring, future researchers can improve the generalizability of their findings by including diverse populations in clinical trials.

Nephrogenic Systemic Fibrosis

Nephrogenic systemic fibrosis (NSF) is an important complication of MR imaging. This disorder was initially recognized in the late 1990s[118] and affects individuals with severe renal dysfunction who receive gadolinium-based contrast agents. Although the prevalence of NSF is low, the disease can be lethal, and hence the use of MR contrast is contraindicated in those with severe renal impairment.[119]

Patients with NSF generally present with symmetric cutaneous lesions that can cause restriction of joint movement. In addition to the skin, gadolinium deposits have been found in the skeletal muscles, myocardium, and

gastrointestinal tract. Whereas the clinical manifestations of NSF have been well described, its pathogenesis is still not well understood, and treatment options have not been well studied.[119] The US Food and Drug Administration

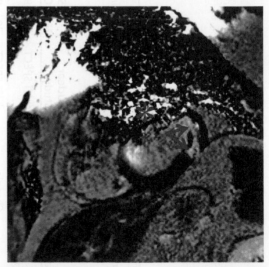

Fig. 17. Left-sided implantable cardioverter-defibrillator generator creates signal loss in the anterior and anteroseptal territory (*asterisk* denotes the artifact). In this LGE image, inferolateral subendocardial infarct can still be seen (*red arrows*).

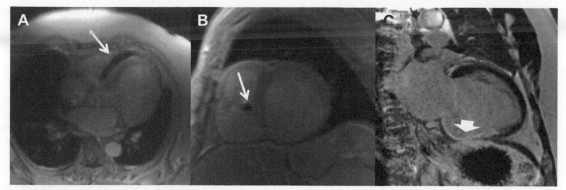

Fig. 18. CMR images of a patient with a right-sided implantable cardioverter-defibrillator generator. (*A*) An axial image showing the signal loss artifact generated by the ventricular implantable cardioverter-defibrillator lead (*long arrow*). (*B*) Short axis image of the lead artifact (*long arrow*). (*C*) The basal inferior subendocardial infarct and the midinferior transmural infarct are well visualized on LGE imaging (*short arrow*).

(FDA) recommends against the administration of gadolinium-based contrast to patients with a glomerular filtration rate less than 30 mL/min/1.7 m².

Implantable Cardioverter-Defibrillator/Pacemaker

The presence of an implanted pacemaker or defibrillator has generally been considered an absolute contraindication to MR imaging. However, recent investigations have reported that MR imaging can be performed without incident in patients with devices in some circumstances, and when appropriate precautions are taken.[120,121] Performing cardiac MR imaging in patients with devices adds additional complexity because the generator and leads may result in artifacts that obscure portions of the heart (**Fig. 17**). Nevertheless, useful information can often be obtained concerning cardiac function and viability (**Fig. 18**).[122]

Position statements from the American Heart Association[123] and European Society of Cardiology[124] note that MR imaging should be considered in patients with devices only when there is a compelling clinical need. Studies should be performed only in experienced centers, with close collaboration between radiology and electrophysiology. Devices should be interrogated before and after the study, and patients should be monitored closely while in the MR imaging system. A new pacemaker system has been approved as MR imaging compatible by the FDA for imaging outside the chest and is being tested for safety in cardiac imaging.[125]

Cost-Effectiveness of CMR Imaging

In a study by Miller and colleagues,[126] 110 patients with chest pain and an intermediate to high probability of CAD were randomized to evaluation with stress cardiac MR in an observation unit or to usual inpatient care. Observation unit management with stress MR decreased cost and did not result in any missed MIs. Data concerning the cost-effectiveness of CMR imaging in other settings are still limited.

SUMMARY

As concerns about exposure to ionizing radiation from diagnostic testing continue to grow,[8] CMR imaging presents a compelling alternative to other cardiac imaging modalities. CMR imaging has superior spatial resolution than echocardiography and SPECT, is competitive with PET, and can be performed safely in most individuals.[9,85] The use of CMR imaging allows for the detection of changes in cardiac perfusion as well as in structure and function, providing incremental prognostic value.[88] As awareness of and access to CMR imaging grow among health care providers, CMR imaging is likely to become an increasingly used and essential component of diagnostic decision making.

REFERENCES

1. Lloyd-Jones D, Adamo RJ, Brown TM, et al. Heart disease and stroke statistics–2010 update: a report from the American Heart Association. Circulation 2010;121(7):e46–215.
2. Greenland P, Alpert JS, Beller GA, et al. 2010 ACCF/AHA guideline for assessment of cardiovascular risk in asymptomatic adults: a report of the American College of Cardiology Foundation/American Heart Association Task Force on Practice Guidelines. J Am Coll Cardiol 2010;56(25):e50–103.

3. Hundley WG, Morgan TM, Neagle CM, et al. Magnetic resonance imaging determination of cardiac prognosis. Circulation 2002;106(18):2328–33.

4. Jahnke C, Nagel E, Gebker R, et al. Prognostic value of cardiac magnetic resonance stress tests: adenosine stress perfusion and dobutamine stress wall motion imaging. Circulation 2007;115(13):1769–76.

5. Schwitter J, Nanz D, Kneifel S, et al. Assessment of myocardial perfusion in coronary artery disease by magnetic resonance: a comparison with positron emission tomography and coronary angiography. Circulation 2001;103(18):2230–5.

6. Schwitter J, Arai AE. Assessment of cardiac ischaemia and viability: role of cardiovascular magnetic resonance. Eur Heart J 2011;32(7):799–809.

7. Cardis E, Vrijheid M, Blettner M, et al. Risk of cancer after low doses of ionising radiation: retrospective cohort study in 15 countries. BMJ 2005;331(7508):77.

8. Fazel R, Krumholz HM, Wang Y, et al. Exposure to low-dose ionizing radiation from medical imaging procedures. N Engl J Med 2009;361(9):849–57.

9. Wagner A, Mahrholdt H, Holly TA, et al. Contrast-enhanced MRI and routine single photon emission computed tomography (SPECT) perfusion imaging for detection of subendocardial myocardial infarcts: an imaging study. Lancet 2003;361(9355):374–9.

10. Beek AM, van Rossum AC. Use of cardiovascular magnetic resonance imaging in the assessment of left ventricular function, scar and viability in patients with ischaemic cardiomyopathy and chronic myocardial infarction. Heart 2010;96(18):1494–501.

11. Kim RJ, Farzaneh-Far A. The diagnostic utility of cardiovascular magnetic resonance in patients with chest pain, elevated cardiac enzymes and non-obstructed coronary arteries. Rev Esp Cardiol 2009;62(9):966–71.

12. Lee VS. Cardiovascular MRI: Physical Principles to Practical Protocols. 1st edition. Philadelphia: Lippincott Williams & Wilkins; 2006.

13. Cerqueira MD, Verani MS, Schwaiger M, et al. Safety profile of adenosine stress perfusion imaging: results from the Adenoscan Multicenter Trial Registry. J Am Coll Cardiol 1994;23(2):384–9.

14. Ricciardi MJ, Wu E, Davidson CJ, et al. Visualization of discrete microinfarction after percutaneous coronary intervention associated with mild creatine kinase-MB elevation. Circulation 2001;103(23):2780–3.

15. Kim RJ, Fieno DS, Parrish TB, et al. Relationship of MRI delayed contrast enhancement to irreversible injury, infarct age, and contractile function. Circulation 1999;100(19):1992–2002.

16. Rehwald WG, Fieno DS, Chen EL, et al. Myocardial magnetic resonance imaging contrast agent concentrations after reversible and irreversible ischemic injury. Circulation 2002;105(2):224–9.

17. Bulow H, Klein C, Kuehn I, et al. Cardiac magnetic resonance imaging: long term reproducibility of the late enhancement signal in patients with chronic coronary artery disease. Heart 2005;91(9):1158–63.

18. Kushner FG, Hand M, Smith SC Jr, et al. 2009 Focused Updates: ACC/AHA Guidelines for the Management of Patients With ST-Elevation Myocardial Infarction (updating the 2004 Guideline and 2007 Focused Update) and ACC/AHA/SCAI Guidelines on Percutaneous Coronary Intervention (updating the 2005 Guideline and 2007 Focused Update): a report of the American College of Cardiology Foundation/American Heart Association Task Force on Practice Guidelines. Circulation 2009;120(22):2271–306.

19. Anderson JL, Adams CD, Antman EM, et al. ACC/AHA 2007 guidelines for the management of patients with unstable angina/non ST-elevation myocardial infarction: a report of the American College of Cardiology/American Heart Association Task Force on Practice Guidelines (Writing Committee to Revise the 2002 Guidelines for the Management of Patients With Unstable Angina/Non ST-Elevation Myocardial Infarction): developed in collaboration with the American College of Emergency Physicians, the Society for Cardiovascular Angiography and Interventions, and the Society of Thoracic Surgeons: endorsed by the American Association of Cardiovascular and Pulmonary Rehabilitation and the Society for Academic Emergency Medicine. Circulation 2007;116(7):e148–304.

20. Amsterdam EA, Kirk JD, Bluemke DA, et al. Testing of low-risk patients presenting to the emergency department with chest pain: a scientific statement from the American Heart Association. Circulation 2010;122(17):1756–76.

21. Assomull RG, Lyne JC, Keenan N, et al. The role of cardiovascular magnetic resonance in patients presenting with chest pain, raised troponin, and unobstructed coronary arteries. Eur Heart J 2007;28(10):1242–9.

22. Kwong RY, Schussheim AE, Rekhraj S, et al. Detecting acute coronary syndrome in the emergency department with cardiac magnetic resonance imaging. Circulation 2003;107(4):531–7.

23. Cury RC, Shash K, Nagurney JT, et al. Cardiac magnetic resonance with T2-weighted imaging improves detection of patients with acute coronary syndrome in the emergency department. Circulation 2008;118(8):837–44.

24. Litmanovich D, Bankier AA, Cantin L, et al. CT and MRI in diseases of the aorta. AJR Am J Roentgenol 2009;193(4):928–40.

25. Abdel-Aty H, Boye P, Zagrosek A, et al. Diagnostic performance of cardiovascular magnetic resonance in patients with suspected acute myocarditis: comparison of different approaches. J Am Coll Cardiol 2005;45(11):1815–22.

26. Eitel I, Behrendt F, Schindler K, et al. Differential diagnosis of suspected apical ballooning syndrome using contrast-enhanced magnetic resonance imaging. Eur Heart J 2008;29(21):2651–9.

27. Wright RS, Anderson JL, Adams CD, et al. 2011 ACCF/AHA focused update of the Guidelines for the Management of Patients with Unstable Angina/Non-ST-Elevation Myocardial Infarction (updating the 2007 guideline): a report of the American College of Cardiology Foundation/American Heart Association Task Force on Practice Guidelines developed in collaboration with the American College of Emergency Physicians, Society for Cardiovascular Angiography and Interventions, and Society of Thoracic Surgeons. J Am Coll Cardiol 2011;57(19):1920–59.

28. Raman SV, Simonetti OP, Winner MW 3rd, et al. Cardiac magnetic resonance with edema imaging identifies myocardium at risk and predicts worse outcome in patients with non-ST-segment elevation acute coronary syndrome. J Am Coll Cardiol 2010; 55(22):2480–8.

29. Kim RJ, Albert TS, Wible JH, et al. Performance of delayed-enhancement magnetic resonance imaging with gadoversetamide contrast for the detection and assessment of myocardial infarction: an international, multicenter, double-blinded, randomized trial. Circulation 2008;117(5):629–37.

30. Abdel-Aty H, Zagrosek A, Schulz-Menger J, et al. Delayed enhancement and T2-weighted cardiovascular magnetic resonance imaging differentiate acute from chronic myocardial infarction. Circulation 2004;109(20):2411–6.

31. Saeed M, Weber O, Lee R, et al. Discrimination of myocardial acute and chronic (scar) infarctions on delayed contrast enhanced magnetic resonance imaging with intravascular magnetic resonance contrast media. J Am Coll Cardiol 2006;48(10): 1961–8.

32. Plein S, Greenwood JP, Ridgway JP, et al. Assessment of non-ST-segment elevation acute coronary syndromes with cardiac magnetic resonance imaging. J Am Coll Cardiol 2004;44(11):2173–81.

33. Hamon M, Agostini D, Le Page O, et al. Prognostic impact of right ventricular involvement in patients with acute myocardial infarction: meta-analysis. Crit Care Med 2008;36(7):2023–33.

34. Kumar A, Abdel-Aty H, Kriedemann I, et al. Contrast-enhanced cardiovascular magnetic resonance imaging of right ventricular infarction. J Am Coll Cardiol 2006;48(10):1969–76.

35. Mollet NR, Dymarkowski S, Volders W, et al. Visualization of ventricular thrombi with contrast-enhanced magnetic resonance imaging in patients with ischemic heart disease. Circulation 2002;106(23): 2873–6.

36. Hombach V, Grebe O, Merkle N, et al. Sequelae of acute myocardial infarction regarding cardiac structure and function and their prognostic significance as assessed by magnetic resonance imaging. Eur Heart J 2005;26(6):549–57.

37. Tanimoto T, Imanishi T, Kitabata H, et al. Prevalence and clinical significance of papillary muscle infarction detected by late gadolinium-enhanced magnetic resonance imaging in patients with ST-segment elevation myocardial infarction. Circulation 2010;122(22):2281–7.

38. Srichai MB, Junor C, Rodriguez LL, et al. Clinical, imaging, and pathological characteristics of left ventricular thrombus: a comparison of contrast-enhanced magnetic resonance imaging, transthoracic echocardiography, and transesophageal echocardiography with surgical or pathological validation. Am Heart J 2006;152(1):75–84.

39. Syed MA, Carlson K, Murphy M, et al. Long-term safety of cardiac magnetic resonance imaging performed in the first few days after bare-metal stent implantation. J Magn Reson Imaging 2006;24(5): 1056–61.

40. Barbier CE, Bjerner T, Johansson L, et al. Myocardial scars more frequent than expected: magnetic resonance imaging detects potential risk group. J Am Coll Cardiol 2006;48(4):765–71.

41. Kim HW, Klem I, Shah DJ, et al. Unrecognized non-Q-wave myocardial infarction: prevalence and prognostic significance in patients with suspected coronary disease. PLoS Med 2009;6(4):e1000057.

42. Ebeling Barbier C, Bjerner T, Hansen T, et al. Clinically unrecognized myocardial infarction detected at MR imaging may not be associated with atherosclerosis. Radiology 2007;245(1):103–10.

43. Kwong RY, Chan AK, Brown KA, et al. Impact of unrecognized myocardial scar detected by cardiac magnetic resonance imaging on event-free survival in patients presenting with signs or symptoms of coronary artery disease. Circulation 2006;113(23): 2733–43.

44. Kwong RY, Sattar H, Wu H, et al. Incidence and prognostic implication of unrecognized myocardial scar characterized by cardiac magnetic resonance in diabetic patients without clinical evidence of myocardial infarction. Circulation 2008;118(10): 1011–20.

45. Ganame J, Messalli G, Dymarkowski S, et al. Impact of myocardial haemorrhage on left ventricular function and remodelling in patients with

reperfused acute myocardial infarction. Eur Heart J 2009;30(12):1440–9.

46. Basso C, Corbetti F, Silva C, et al. Morphologic validation of reperfused hemorrhagic myocardial infarction by cardiovascular magnetic resonance. Am J Cardiol 2007;100(8):1322–7.

47. O'Regan DP, Ahmed R, Karunanithy N, et al. Reperfusion hemorrhage following acute myocardial infarction: assessment with T2* mapping and effect on measuring the area at risk. Radiology 2009; 250(3):916–22.

48. Eitel I, Kubusch K, Strohm O, et al. Prognostic value and determinants of a hypointense infarct core in T2-weighted cardiac magnetic resonance in acute reperfused ST-elevation myocardial infarction. Circ Cardiovasc Imaging 2011;4(4): 354–62.

49. Fieno DS, Kim RJ, Chen EL, et al. Contrast-enhanced magnetic resonance imaging of myocardium at risk: distinction between reversible and irreversible injury throughout infarct healing. J Am Coll Cardiol 2000;36(6):1985–91.

50. Ito H, Maruyama A, Iwakura K, et al. Clinical implications of the 'no reflow' phenomenon. A predictor of complications and left ventricular remodeling in reperfused anterior wall myocardial infarction. Circulation 1996;93(2):223–8.

51. Wu KC, Zerhouni EA, Judd RM, et al. Prognostic significance of microvascular obstruction by magnetic resonance imaging in patients with acute myocardial infarction. Circulation 1998;97(8): 765–72.

52. Nijveldt R, Beek AM, Hirsch A, et al. Functional recovery after acute myocardial infarction: comparison between angiography, electrocardiography, and cardiovascular magnetic resonance measures of microvascular injury. J Am Coll Cardiol 2008; 52(3):181–9.

53. de Waha S, Desch S, Eitel I, et al. Impact of early vs. late microvascular obstruction assessed by magnetic resonance imaging on long-term outcome after ST-elevation myocardial infarction: a comparison with traditional prognostic markers. Eur Heart J 2010;31(21):2660–8.

54. Gibbons RJ, Miller TD, Christian TF. Infarct size measured by single photon emission computed tomographic imaging with (99m)Tc-sestamibi: a measure of the efficacy of therapy in acute myocardial infarction. Circulation 2000;101(1): 101–8.

55. Eitel I, Desch S, Fuernau G, et al. Prognostic significance and determinants of myocardial salvage assessed by cardiovascular magnetic resonance in acute reperfused myocardial infarction. J Am Coll Cardiol 2010;55(22):2470–9.

56. Beek AM, Kuhl HP, Bondarenko O, et al. Delayed contrast-enhanced magnetic resonance imaging for the prediction of regional functional improvement after acute myocardial infarction. J Am Coll Cardiol 2003;42(5):895–901.

57. Gerber BL, Garot J, Bluemke DA, et al. Accuracy of contrast-enhanced magnetic resonance imaging in predicting improvement of regional myocardial function in patients after acute myocardial infarction. Circulation 2002;106(9):1083–9.

58. Choi KM, Kim RJ, Gubernikoff G, et al. Transmural extent of acute myocardial infarction predicts long-term improvement in contractile function. Circulation 2001;104(10):1101–7.

59. Huang BS, Leenen FH. The brain renin-angiotensin-aldosterone system: a major mechanism for sympathetic hyperactivity and left ventricular remodeling and dysfunction after myocardial infarction. Curr Heart Fail Rep 2009;6(2):81–8.

60. Masci PG, Ganame J, Strata E, et al. Myocardial salvage by CMR correlates with LV remodeling and early ST-segment resolution in acute myocardial infarction. JACC Cardiovasc Imaging 2010; 3(1):45–51.

61. Lund GK, Stork A, Muellerleile K, et al. Prediction of left ventricular remodeling and analysis of infarct resorption in patients with reperfused myocardial infarcts by using contrast-enhanced MR imaging. Radiology 2007;245(1):95–102.

62. Nijveldt R, Hofman MB, Hirsch A, et al. Assessment of microvascular obstruction and prediction of short-term remodeling after acute myocardial infarction: cardiac MR imaging study. Radiology 2009;250(2):363–70.

63. Mammen L, White RD, Woodard PK, et al. ACR Appropriateness Criteria® on chest pain, suggestive of acute coronary syndrome. J Am Coll Radiol 2011;8(1):12–8.

64. O'Neil B, Peacock WF. Cardiac computed tomography in the rapid evaluation of acute cardiac emergencies. Rev Cardiovasc Med 2010;11(Suppl 2): S35–44.

65. Klein C, Nekolla SG, Bengel FM, et al. Assessment of myocardial viability with contrast-enhanced magnetic resonance imaging: comparison with positron emission tomography. Circulation 2002; 105(2):162–7.

66. Hillenbrand HB, Kim RJ, Parker MA, et al. Early assessment of myocardial salvage by contrast-enhanced magnetic resonance imaging. Circulation 2000;102(14):1678–83.

67. Wu E, Ortiz JT, Tejedor P, et al. Infarct size by contrast enhanced cardiac magnetic resonance is a stronger predictor of outcomes than left ventricular ejection fraction or end-systolic volume index: prospective cohort study. Heart 2008; 94(6):730–6.

68. Plein S, Kozerke S, Suerder D, et al. High spatial resolution myocardial perfusion cardiac magnetic

resonance for the detection of coronary artery disease. Eur Heart J 2008;29(17):3148–56.

69. Nagel E, Klein C, Paetsch I, et al. Magnetic resonance perfusion measurements for the noninvasive detection of coronary artery disease. Circulation 2003;108(4):432–7.

70. Ishida N, Sakuma H, Motoyasu M, et al. Noninfarcted myocardium: correlation between dynamic first-pass contrast-enhanced myocardial MR imaging and quantitative coronary angiography. Radiology 2003;229(1):209–16.

71. Kitagawa K, Sakuma H, Nagata M, et al. Diagnostic accuracy of stress myocardial perfusion MRI and late gadolinium-enhanced MRI for detecting flow-limiting coronary artery disease: a multicenter study. Eur Radiol 2008;18(12):2808–16.

72. Schwitter J, Wacker CM, van Rossum AC, et al. MR-IMPACT: comparison of perfusion-cardiac magnetic resonance with single-photon emission computed tomography for the detection of coronary artery disease in a multicentre, multivendor, randomized trial. Eur Heart J 2008; 29(4):480–9.

73. Sakuma H, Suzawa N, Ichikawa Y, et al. Diagnostic accuracy of stress first-pass contrast-enhanced myocardial perfusion MRI compared with stress myocardial perfusion scintigraphy. AJR Am J Roentgenol 2005;185(1):95–102.

74. Lockie T, Ishida M, Perera D, et al. High-resolution magnetic resonance myocardial perfusion imaging at 3.0-Tesla to detect hemodynamically significant coronary stenoses as determined by fractional flow reserve. J Am Coll Cardiol 2011;57(1):70–5.

75. Bodi V, Sanchis J, Lopez-Lereu MP, et al. Prognostic value of dipyridamole stress cardiovascular magnetic resonance imaging in patients with known or suspected coronary artery disease. J Am Coll Cardiol 2007;50(12):1174–9.

76. Krittayaphong R, Chaithiraphan V, Maneesai A, et al. Prognostic value of combined magnetic resonance myocardial perfusion imaging and late gadolinium enhancement. Int J Cardiovasc Imaging 2011;27(5):705–14.

77. Nandalur KR, Dwamena BA, Choudhri AF, et al. Diagnostic performance of stress cardiac magnetic resonance imaging in the detection of coronary artery disease: a meta-analysis. J Am Coll Cardiol 2007;50(14):1343–53.

78. Ingkanisorn WP, Kwong RY, Bohme NS, et al. Prognosis of negative adenosine stress magnetic resonance in patients presenting to an emergency department with chest pain. J Am Coll Cardiol 2006;47(7):1427–32.

79. Nagel E, Lehmkuhl HB, Bocksch W, et al. Noninvasive diagnosis of ischemia-induced wall motion abnormalities with the use of high-dose dobutamine stress MRI: comparison with dobutamine stress echocardiography. Circulation 1999;99(6): 763–70.

80. Gebker R, Jahnke C, Hucko T, et al. Dobutamine stress magnetic resonance imaging for the detection of coronary artery disease in women. Heart 2010;96(8):616–20.

81. Paetsch I, Jahnke C, Ferrari VA, et al. Determination of interobserver variability for identifying inducible left ventricular wall motion abnormalities during dobutamine stress magnetic resonance imaging. Eur Heart J 2006;27(12):1459–64.

82. Hundley WG, Hamilton CA, Thomas MS, et al. Utility of fast cine magnetic resonance imaging and display for the detection of myocardial ischemia in patients not well suited for second harmonic stress echocardiography. Circulation 1999;100(16):1697–702.

83. Schalla S, Klein C, Paetsch I, et al. Real-time MR image acquisition during high-dose dobutamine hydrochloride stress for detecting left ventricular wall-motion abnormalities in patients with coronary arterial disease. Radiology 2002; 224(3):845–51.

84. Rerkpattanapipat P, Gandhi SK, Darty SN, et al. Feasibility to detect severe coronary artery stenoses with upright treadmill exercise magnetic resonance imaging. Am J Cardiol 2003;92(5):603–6.

85. Wahl A, Paetsch I, Gollesch A, et al. Safety and feasibility of high-dose dobutamine-atropine stress cardiovascular magnetic resonance for diagnosis of myocardial ischaemia: experience in 1000 consecutive cases. Eur Heart J 2004;25(14): 1230–6.

86. Syed MA, Paterson DI, Ingkanisorn WP, et al. Reproducibility and inter-observer variability of dobutamine stress CMR in patients with severe coronary disease: implications for clinical research. J Cardiovasc Magn Reson 2005;7(5):763–8.

87. Gebker R, Jahnke C, Manka R, et al. Additional value of myocardial perfusion imaging during dobutamine stress magnetic resonance for the assessment of coronary artery disease. Circ Cardiovasc Imaging 2008;1(2):122–30.

88. Bingham SE, Hachamovitch R. Incremental prognostic significance of combined cardiac magnetic resonance imaging, adenosine stress perfusion, delayed enhancement, and left ventricular function over preimaging information for the prediction of adverse events. Circulation 2011;123(14):1509–18.

89. Raman SV, Dickerson JA, Jekic M, et al. Real-time cine and myocardial perfusion with treadmill exercise stress cardiovascular magnetic resonance in patients referred for stress SPECT. J Cardiovasc Magn Reson 2010;12:41.

90. Sakuma H. Coronary CT versus MR angiography: the role of MR angiography. Radiology 2011; 258(2):340–9.

91. Kim WY, Danias PG, Stuber M, et al. Coronary magnetic resonance angiography for the detection of coronary stenoses. N Engl J Med 2001;345(26): 1863–9.

92. Jahnke C, Paetsch I, Nehrke K, et al. Rapid and complete coronary arterial tree visualization with magnetic resonance imaging: feasibility and diagnostic performance. Eur Heart J 2005;26(21): 2313–9.

93. Sakuma H, Ichikawa Y, Chino S, et al. Detection of coronary artery stenosis with whole-heart coronary magnetic resonance angiography. J Am Coll Cardiol 2006;48(10):1946–50.

94. Cheng AS, Pegg TJ, Karamitsos TD, et al. Cardiovascular magnetic resonance perfusion imaging at 3-tesla for the detection of coronary artery disease: a comparison with 1.5-tesla. J Am Coll Cardiol 2007;49(25):2440–9.

95. Hu P, Chan J, Ngo LH, et al. Contrast-enhanced whole-heart coronary MRI with bolus infusion of gadobenate dimeglumine at 1.5 T. Magn Reson Med 2011;65(2):392–8.

96. Selvanayagam JB, Jerosch-Herold M, Porto I, et al. Resting myocardial blood flow is impaired in hibernating myocardium: a magnetic resonance study of quantitative perfusion assessment. Circulation 2005;112(21):3289–96.

97. Kelle S, Hays AG, Hirsch GA, et al. Coronary artery distensibility assessed by 3.0 tesla coronary magnetic resonance imaging in subjects with and without coronary artery disease. Am J Cardiol 2011;108(4):491–7.

98. Tillisch J, Brunken R, Marshall R, et al. Reversibility of cardiac wall-motion abnormalities predicted by positron tomography. N Engl J Med 1986;314(14): 884–8.

99. Bax JJ, Poldermans D, Elhendy A, et al. Sensitivity, specificity, and predictive accuracies of various noninvasive techniques for detecting hibernating myocardium. Curr Probl Cardiol 2001;26(2): 147–86.

100. Meluzin J, Cerny J, Frelich M, et al. Prognostic value of the amount of dysfunctional but viable myocardium in revascularized patients with coronary artery disease and left ventricular dysfunction. Investigators of this Multicenter Study. J Am Coll Cardiol 1998;32(4):912–20.

101. Pagley PR, Beller GA, Watson DD, et al. Improved outcome after coronary bypass surgery in patients with ischemic cardiomyopathy and residual myocardial viability. Circulation 1997;96(3):793–800.

102. Klocke FJ, Baird MG, Lorell BH, et al. ACC/AHA/ASNC guidelines for the clinical use of cardiac radionuclide imaging–executive summary: a report of the American College of Cardiology/American Heart Association Task Force on Practice Guidelines (ACC/AHA/ASNC Committee to Revise the 1995 Guidelines for the Clinical Use of Cardiac Radionuclide Imaging). Circulation 2003;108(11): 1404–18.

103. Kim RJ, Wu E, Rafael A, et al. The use of contrast-enhanced magnetic resonance imaging to identify reversible myocardial dysfunction. N Engl J Med 2000;343(20):1445–53.

104. Gutberlet M, Frohlich M, Mehl S, et al. Myocardial viability assessment in patients with highly impaired left ventricular function: comparison of delayed enhancement, dobutamine stress MRI, end-diastolic wall thickness, and Tl201-SPECT with functional recovery after revascularization. Eur Radiol 2005;15(5):872–80.

105. Kitagawa K, Sakuma H, Hirano T, et al. Acute myocardial infarction: myocardial viability assessment in patients early thereafter comparison of contrast-enhanced MR imaging with resting (201) Tl SPECT. Single photon emission computed tomography. Radiology 2003;226(1):138–44.

106. Kuhl HP, Beek AM, van der Weerdt AP, et al. Myocardial viability in chronic ischemic heart disease: comparison of contrast-enhanced magnetic resonance imaging with (18)F-fluorodeoxyglucose positron emission tomography. J Am Coll Cardiol 2003; 41(8):1341–8.

107. Kuhl HP, Lipke CS, Krombach GA, et al. Assessment of reversible myocardial dysfunction in chronic ischaemic heart disease: comparison of contrast-enhanced cardiovascular magnetic resonance and a combined positron emission tomography-single photon emission computed tomography imaging protocol. Eur Heart J 2006; 27(7):846–53.

108. Wu YW, Tadamura E, Yamamuro M, et al. Comparison of contrast-enhanced MRI with (18)F-FDG PET/201Tl SPECT in dysfunctional myocardium: relation to early functional outcome after surgical revascularization in chronic ischemic heart disease. J Nucl Med 2007;48(7):1096–103.

109. Knuesel PR, Nanz D, Wyss C, et al. Characterization of dysfunctional myocardium by positron emission tomography and magnetic resonance: relation to functional outcome after revascularization. Circulation 2003;108(9):1095–100.

110. Baer FM, Theissen P, Crnac J, et al. Head to head comparison of dobutamine-transoesophageal echocardiography and dobutamine-magnetic resonance imaging for the prediction of left ventricular functional recovery in patients with chronic coronary artery disease. Eur Heart J 2000;21(12): 981–91.

111. Schinkel AF, Bax JJ, Poldermans D, et al. Hibernating myocardium: diagnosis and patient outcomes. Curr Probl Cardiol 2007;32(7):375–410.

112. Bristow MR, Saxon LA, Boehmer J, et al. Cardiac-resynchronization therapy with or without an

implantable defibrillator in advanced chronic heart failure. N Engl J Med 2004;350(21):2140–50.

113. Ypenburg C, Schalij MJ, Bleeker GB, et al. Impact of viability and scar tissue on response to cardiac resynchronization therapy in ischaemic heart failure patients. Eur Heart J 2007;28(1):33–41.

114. Bleeker GB, Kaandorp TA, Lamb HJ, et al. Effect of posterolateral scar tissue on clinical and echocardiographic improvement after cardiac resynchronization therapy. Circulation 2006;113(7):969–76.

115. Leyva F, Foley PW, Chalil S, et al. Cardiac resynchronisation therapy guided by late gadolinium-enhancement cardiovascular magnetic resonance. J Cardiovasc Magn Reson 2011;13(1):29.

116. Nezafat R, Han Y, Peters DC, et al. Coronary magnetic resonance vein imaging: imaging contrast, sequence, and timing. Magn Reson Med 2007;58(6):1196–206.

117. Sievers B, Elliott MD, Hurwitz LM, et al. Rapid detection of myocardial infarction by subsecond, free-breathing delayed contrast-enhancement cardiovascular magnetic resonance. Circulation 2007;115(2):236–44.

118. Cowper SE, Robin HS, Steinberg SM, et al. Scleromyxoedema-like cutaneous diseases in renal-dialysis patients. Lancet 2000;356(9234):1000–1.

119. Kribben A, Witzke O, Hillen U, et al. Nephrogenic systemic fibrosis: pathogenesis, diagnosis, and therapy. J Am Coll Cardiol 2009;53(18):1621–8.

120. Sommer T, Naehle CP, Yang A, et al. Strategy for safe performance of extrathoracic magnetic resonance imaging at 1.5 tesla in the presence of cardiac pacemakers in non-pacemaker-dependent patients: a prospective study with 115 examinations. Circulation 2006;114(12):1285–92.

121. Naehle CP, Strach K, Thomas D, et al. Magnetic resonance imaging at 1.5-T in patients with implantable cardioverter-defibrillators. J Am Coll Cardiol 2009;54(6):549–55.

122. Nazarian S, Roguin A, Zviman MM, et al. Clinical utility and safety of a protocol for noncardiac and cardiac magnetic resonance imaging of patients with permanent pacemakers and implantable-cardioverter defibrillators at 1.5 tesla. Circulation 2006;114(12):1277–84.

123. Levine GN, Gomes AS, Arai AE, et al. Safety of magnetic resonance imaging in patients with cardiovascular devices: an American Heart Association scientific statement from the Committee on Diagnostic and Interventional Cardiac Catheterization, Council on Clinical Cardiology, and the Council on Cardiovascular Radiology and Intervention: endorsed by the American College of Cardiology Foundation, the North American Society for Cardiac Imaging, and the Society for Cardiovascular Magnetic Resonance. Circulation 2007; 116(24):2878–91.

124. Roguin A, Schwitter J, Vahlhaus C, et al. Magnetic resonance imaging in individuals with cardiovascular implantable electronic devices. Europace 2008;10(3):336–46.

125. Wilkoff BL, Bello D, Taborsky M, et al. Magnetic resonance imaging in patients with a pacemaker system designed for the magnetic resonance environment. Heart Rhythm 2011;8(1):65–73.

126. Miller CD, Hwang W, Hoekstra JW, et al. Stress cardiac magnetic resonance imaging with observation unit care reduces cost for patients with emergent chest pain: a randomized trial. Ann Emerg Med 2010;56(3):209–19, e202.

MR Imaging of Nonischemic Cardiomyopathy

Saurabh Jha, MBBS[a],*, Ari Goldberg, MD, PhD[b],
Mark Stellingworth, MD[c]

KEYWORDS

- Cardiac MR imaging • Nonischemic cardiomyopathy
- Coronary artery disease

Cardiomyopathy, or failing heart, is broadly divided into ischemic and nonischemic cardiomyopathy. The term ischemic technically includes processes at the macrocirculatory and microcirculatory level. However, ischemic cardiomyopathy for the purposes of this review refers to myocardial dysfunction due to coronary artery disease (CAD), and does not include entities that cause primary or secondary dysfunction solely of the microcirculation. The most common cause of CAD is atherosclerosis.[1]

Nonischemic cardiomyopathy represents an assortment of disorders whose common primary defining character is the absence of a causative link with CAD. While broad-based, this distinction is important because it affects management. Ischemic cardiomyopathy is potentially remediable by revascularization (coronary artery bypass graft and/or percutaneous coronary interventions). The treatment of nonischemic cardiomyopathy focuses on the cause, and often the only treatment is heart transplantation.

Cardiac magnetic resonance imaging (CMR) interrogates the heart with a high spatial, temporal, and soft-tissue resolution, and multiplanar capability. It is able to quantify flow and function in a manner at least comparable to echocardiography. CMR is not plagued by technical factors that afflict echo such as the degree of operator dependency, patient body habitus, and coexisting pathology such as chronic airflow limitation[2]; this means that CMR, at least in terms of quantification, is more reproducible than echo.[3] Due to the complex geometry of the right ventricle, CMR is able to interrogate this structure with far greater clarity than echocardiography.[4] However, the uniqueness of CMR lies not in its ability to surpass echo in quantification, but to provide distinction of tissue types, the most important being myocardium that has sustained injury. This appearance is referred to as scar imaging or late gadolinium enhancement (LGE).[5]

LATE GADOLINIUM ENHANCEMENT

LGE is a feature of injured myocardium. The injury may be acute or chronic.[5] The pattern of scar facilitates the distinction of ischemic from nonischemic cardiomyopathy (**Fig. 1**).[6]

Injured myocardium is detected by the principles of inversion recovery in magnetic resonance (MR) imaging. In brief, application of an inversion pulse flips the longitudinal magnetization from its $+Mz$ resting state to $-Mz$ state, or a similar magnitude but negative polarity. Thereafter, the longitudinal magnetization begins to recover. The rate of recovery is proportional to the T1 recovery time of the tissue, an inherent property of the tissue. Tissues with shorter T1 recover their longitudinal magnetization sooner than tissue with longer T1. Regardless of the recovery time, each tissue crosses a so-called null point. The null point

[a] Department of Radiology, University of Pennsylvania Medical Center, 3400 Spruce Street, Philadelphia, PA 19104, USA
[b] Geisinger Health System, 100 North Academy Avenue, Danville, PA 17822, USA
[c] University Medical Center, 2390 West Congress, Lafayette, LA 70506, USA
* Corresponding author.
E-mail address: saurabh.jha@uphs.upenn.edu

PET Clin 6 (2011) 475–487
doi:10.1016/j.cpet.2011.09.003

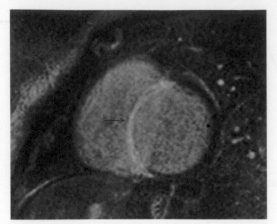

Fig. 1. Inversion recovery obtained 15 minutes after the injection of gadolinium (scar imaging) in the short-axis plane shows septal wall displaying late gadolinium enhancement (LGE) representing scar (*large arrow*), whereas the lateral wall is dark or nulled normal myocardium (*small arrow*). The LGE is transmural, that is, it involves the entire thickness of the myocardium and is territorial. Territorial means that the distribution of the LGE corresponds to coronary artery territory.

is the time point after the inversion pulse when the tissue has no net longitudinal magnetization.[7]

The time taken for the tissue to cross the null point is its unique inversion time (TI). If a pulse is applied at the TI, the nulled tissue fails to emanate signal and is said to be suppressed. The TI is, of course, dependent on the tissue's T1. Fat has a shorter TI than water because of its shorter T1. Thus, inversion recovery is a method of tissue suppression. Pulse sequences employing inversion recovery include STIR (short-tau inversion recovery) and FLAIR (fluid-attenuation inversion recovery) for the suppression of fat and water, respectively.

In scar imaging, inversion recovery suppresses the normal myocardium (**Fig. 2**). The scar appears bright, giving rise to the oft-quoted phrase in the cardiac MR imaging community "bright is dead." Normal myocardium takes up gadolinium sooner than scar and releases the gadolinium before scar. Stated differently, gadolinium is retained by the scar tissue longer than normal myocardium. At a certain time after the injection of gadolinium the difference in the quantity of retained gadolinium between normal myocardium and scar is maximal, and, if the normal myocardium is nulled the contrast between scar and normal myocardium is optimal.

MYOCARDIAL EDEMA

Myocardial edema indicates an acute process and does not per se distinguish between ischemic and nonischemic entities (**Fig. 3**). However, the pattern

of edema may point to a nonischemic entity if it is patchy and nonterritorial in distribution. Myocardial edema is detected by fluid-sensitive sequences such as triple inversion recovery, in which both blood and fat are suppressed.[8]

PATTERN OF LATE GADOLINIUM ENHANCEMENT

The pattern of LGE distinguishes between ischemic cardiomyopathy and nonischemic entities.[9] The pattern of LGE depends on its distribution, mural extent, and morphology. The mural extent may be subendocardial, midmyocardial, subepicardial, or transmural, depending on the portion of the myocardium involved. The distribution may be diffuse, territorial, or nonterritorial. The territorial distribution corresponds to an area subtended by a coronary artery with sharp demarcation. A nonterritorial distribution may be focal or multifocal, without appreciation of anatomic borders defined by blood supply. The morphology of the LGE may be linear or patchy.

Ischemic cardiomyopathy tends to have LGE with a territorial distribution (see **Fig. 1**; **Fig. 4**). The LGE may be subendocardial or transmural. Because the subendocardial layer of the myocardium is most prone to ischemia, sparing of the subendocardium suggests a nonischemic cause.

The LGE pattern caused by nonischemic insults may be subepicardial or midmyocardial. Less likely nonischemic entities may cause a transmural or subendocardial pattern. Diffuse symmetric LGE is more likely to be due to a nonischemic cause. Multifocal LGE not obeying vascular territories also points to a nonischemic cause.

CARDIAC MR IMAGING AND DECISION MAKING

CMR through LGE is both diagnostic and prognostic, with the following applications:

a. Distinction between ischemic and nonischemic cardiomyopathy
b. Search for a specific nonischemic etiology
c. Search for a potential arrhythmogenic focus
d. Prognostication patients
e. Guiding biopsy.

The distinction between ischemic and nonischemic cardiomyopathy is, of course, important for the subsequent management (**Fig. 5**). If the cardiac MR imaging is incorporated early enough in the diagnostic algorithm of a patient with heart failure of unknown etiology, and the pattern of LGE suggests a nonischemic cause, then a diagnostic catheter angiogram may be forgone. Such a candidate for

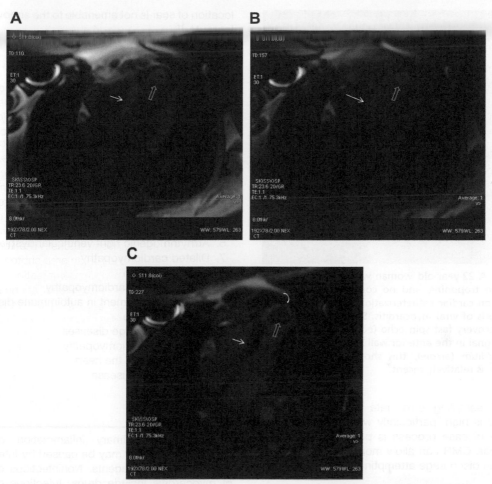

Fig. 2. The principle of inversion recovery for scar imaging is demonstrated with increasing inversion times. Note that the normal myocardium (*white arrow*) initially displays high signal (*A*) then begins to lose signal (*B*) until it is suppressed (*C*). There is some loss in signal of the left ventricular (LV) apical thrombus (*blue arrow*). However, LV apical scar follows a reverse (*curved arrow*) order where it is dark initially and then is bright when the normal myocardium is nulled (*C*).

CMR before catheter angiography may be an individual who fulfills demographic criteria in which there is a very low prevalence of CAD, such as young age or a coexisting systemic pathology that has cardiac manifestations. Sometimes ischemic and nonischemic entities coexist, and CMR may allow clarification of their relative contributions, thereby predicting the return of function with revascularization.

There are findings characteristic of certain entities, and if a high index of suspicion is held, CMR may lead to a specific diagnosis. Even when operating in a clinical vacuum, CMR may strongly suggest a certain diagnosis or allow the imager to offer a limited differential diagnosis.

In patients with both ischemic[10] and nonischemic cardiomyopathy[11] and intractable ventricular arrhythmias, LGE may locate the site for arrhythmogenic focus and ablation, which could reduce procedure time dramatically. If the LGE is midmyocardial or subepicardial and is not accessible to conventional endocardial catheter techniques, this changes the management strategy and is valuable information for the electrophysiologist.

The mere presence of LGE is an independent risk marker for sudden death in many nonischemic cardiomyopathies.[12] The extent of LGE has been shown to correlate negatively with survival in patients with hypertrophic obstructive cardiomyopathy (HOCM).[13] The extent and distribution of LGE determines success of cardiac resynchronization therapy.[14] The presence of LGE aids in the decision toward placement of a prophylactic implantable cardioverter-defibrillator (ICD).[15]

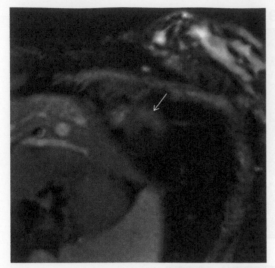

Fig. 3. A 22-year-old woman with acute chest pain, positive troponins, and no coronary artery disease (CAD) on cardiac catheterization with a presumptive diagnosis of viral myocarditis. Short-axis triple-inversion recovery fast spin echo (edema imaging) shows high signal in the anterior wall indicating edematous myocardium (*arrow*); this shows that the disease process is relatively recent.

The sampling error rate of endomyocardial biopsy is high, particularly when the distribution of the disease process is patchy. By localizing the scar, CMR can allow more targeted biopsies or even discourage attempting biopsies when the

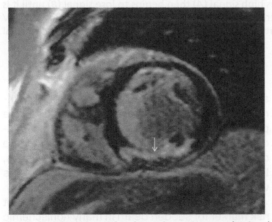

Fig. 4. Scar imaging using inversion recovery obtained 15 minutes after the injection of intravenous gadolinium in the short-axis plane shows LGE of the inferior wall, which is territorial and involves the subendocardial and midmyocardial layers (*arrow*). Given its territorial distribution and involvement of the subendocardial layer of the myocardium, this is an ischemic pattern. The patient had occlusion of the dominant right coronary artery.

location of scar is not amenable to the endovascular route.[16]

NONISCHEMIC DISEASES OF THE HEART

The nonischemic entities to be discussed are listed here. Examples include diseases based on their etiology (sarcoidosis), morphology (dilated cardiomyopathy), and pathogenesis (excessive iron deposition).

1. Viral myocarditis
2. Cardiac sarcoid
3. Cardiac amyloid
4. Eosinophilic heart disease
5. Hypertrophic cardiomyopathy
6. Arrhythmogenic right ventricular dysplasia
7. Dilated cardiomyopathy
8. Noncompaction
9. Drug-induced cardiomyopathy
10. Cardiac involvement in autoimmune diseases
11. Chagas disease
12. Metabolic storage diseases
13. Takatsubo cardiomyopathy
14. Iron overload in the heart
15. Valvular heart disease.

Viral Myocarditis

Myocarditis is primary inflammation of the myocardium, which may be caused by infectious and noninfectious agents. Noninfectious causes of myocarditis include drugs. Infectious causes include bacteria, viruses, and protozoans.

Viral myocarditis is by far the most common cause of myocarditis and, indeed, of an acute nonischemic insult. The LGE is typically subepicardial or midmyocardial in location, affects the basal lateral wall or septal wall, and has a linear morphology.[17] Although this pattern is suggestive of viral myocarditis, it is neither pathognomonic of viral myocarditis nor the only pattern of scar that myocarditis displays. Nonetheless, in a young patient with acute chest pain, elevated troponin, and no evidence of CAD on catheter angiography, if CMR shows this pattern and there is no systemic disease, viral myocarditis should be the first on the differential (**Fig. 6**). About one-third of cases of viral myocarditis progress to dilated cardiomyopathy, and one-third recover.

Sarcoidosis

Sarcoidosis is a multisystem disorder characterized pathologically by noncaseating granulomas. Cardiac involvement was once thought to be infrequent. However, autopsy specimens suggest

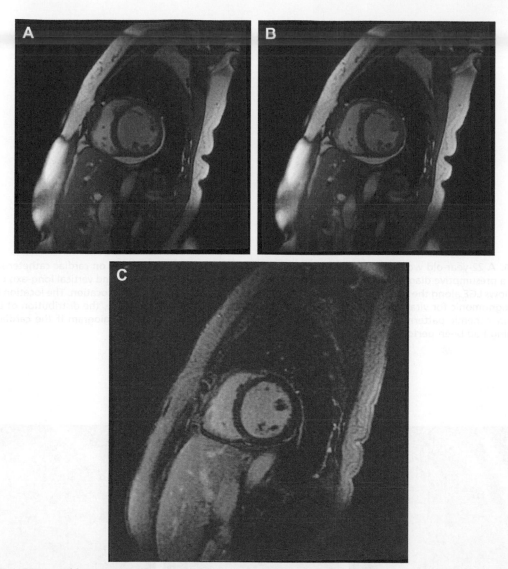

Fig. 5. A 30-year-old man with dyspnea. Still frames from short-axis cine images in end diastole (*A*) and end systole (*B*) show a severely and globally hypokinetic and dilated left ventricle with an ejection fraction of less than 15%. The possibility of CAD was entertained. Scar imaging showed no LGE (*C*). It is unlikely for CAD to cause such severe dysfunction in the absence of scar. The patient subsequently had cardiac catheterization, which confirmed the absence of CAD.

clinically silent cardiac involvement in sarcoidosis with involvement in 20% to 30% of specimens.[18]

Cardiac sarcoid presents with chest pain, heart failure, and arrhythmias. Myocardial edema may be seen in acute cardiac sarcoid. Cardiac sarcoid is more readily detected by scar imaging.[19] The pattern of LGE in cardiac sarcoid has much overlap with myocarditis. However, cardiac sarcoid is typically described as multifocal, patchy, and polymorphic (**Fig. 7**). Even when polymorphic, a nodular pattern is almost exclusively limited to cardiac sarcoid, and is the imaging equivalent of the granulomatous pattern of involvement. The

mural extent of LGE is midmyocardial and subepicardial, as in other nonischemic cardiomyopathies. However, sarcoid can also lead to subendocardial and transmural LGE. Such mural patterns are, of course, more typically associated with CAD, and the question of sarcoid is raised if the distribution is nonterritorial (patchy, multifocal, nonregional). Sarcoid can lead to nonischemic mural patterns of the anterior, apical, and anteroseptal walls.

In a patient with known extracardiac sarcoid, a nonischemic LGE pattern is highly suggestive of cardiac sarcoid. However, in a patient who is

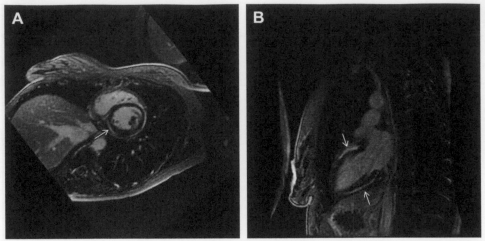

Fig. 6. A 22-year-old woman with acute chest pain, positive troponins, and no CAD on cardiac catheterization with a presumptive diagnosis of viral myocarditis. Scar imaging in the short-axis (*A*) and vertical long-axis planes (*B*) shows LGE along the inferior and anterior walls (*arrow*), which has a subepicardial location. The location is not pathognomonic for viral myocarditis but supports a clinical diagnosis. Of importance, the distribution of LGE is not an ischemic pattern, and the patient might not have needed the catheter angiogram if the cardiac MR imaging had been performed early on.

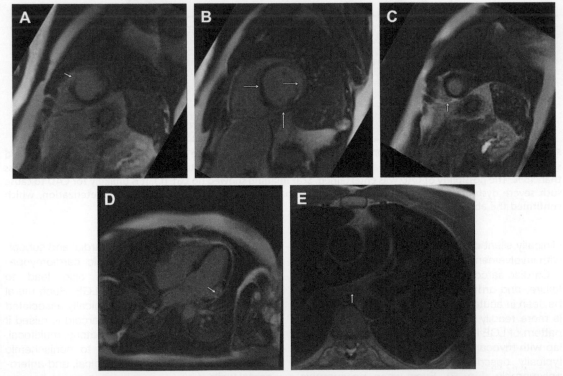

Fig. 7. Scar imaging in the short-axis (*A–C*) and 4-chamber (*D*) planes shows multifocal LGE (*arrows*) that is mid-myocardial (*A, B*) and transmural (*C, D*) affecting the right ventricle as well (*D*). The patient is known to have pulmonary sarcoid and this makes the LGE most likely to be due to cardiac sarcoid. Axial dark blood image (*E*) shows mediastinal adenopathy.

not known to have extracardiac sarcoid, the answer is far from clear cut. Cardiac sarcoid can be the first manifestation of sarcoidosis. However, the sensitivity and specificity of any nonischemic pattern for the diagnosis of sarcoid in the absence of known sarcoid is not known.

Amyloidosis

Amyloidosis may be primary or secondary. Cardiac amyloid portends substantially declining prognostic optimism in sufferers of this truly systemic and protean illness.[20] Cardiac amyloid is a cause of restrictive cardiomyopathy. The mechanism of heart failure is attributable to a diastolic dysfunction, with systolic dysfunction occurring much later in the course of the disease. The importance of diagnosis of cardiac amyloid, despite being imminently untreatable, is the exclusion from other potentially treatable causes of restrictive cardiomyopathy.

MR imaging has proved to be valuable in the diagnosis of cardiac amyloid. The LGE pattern is diffuse and weak in intensity (**Fig. 8**), with a poor contrast between the suppressed myocardium and blood pool. Another way of stating the latter

is that it is difficult to null the myocardium without nulling the blood pool. The reason postulated is that the amyloid binds to the gadolinium, reducing its effective volume of distribution.[21] In addition, T1 mapping post gadolinium can identify myocardium with amyloid deposition.

Amyloidosis leads to thickening of the interatrial septum, valves, and myocardium. The degree of myocardial contraction is less than expected from the degree of wall thickening. Pleural and pericardial effusion will also be captured on MR imaging. In isolation, none of these findings are specific for amyloid, but together and in concert with the findings on LGE would support a clinical diagnosis of amyloid.

Eosinophilic Heart Disease

Eosinophilic myocarditis is part of the hypereosinophilic syndrome. Cardiac involvement leads to heart failure, arrhythmias, and thromboembolism. The heart failure is predominantly caused by diastolic dysfunction and is thus a restrictive cardiomyopathy.

The LGE pattern is typically subendocardial, but with a more global distribution than ischemia if the

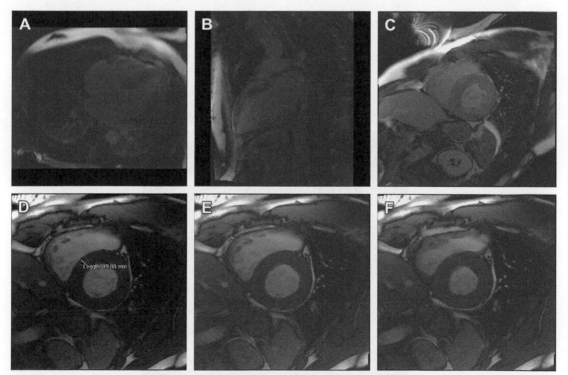

Fig. 8. A 42-year-old man with progressive dyspnea. Scar imaging in the axial (*A*), vertical long-axis (*B*), and short-axis planes (*C*) shows a weak diffuse enhancement of the myocardium, a finding that can be seen in cardiac amyloid. The LV myocardium is thickened (*D*). The still frames of short-axis cine images in end diastole (*E*) and end systole (*F*) show a dysfunctional left ventricle. The ejection fraction is 34%. The patient had an endomyocardial biopsy that showed cardiac amyloid.

inflammation is centered in the endomyocardium. The LGE pattern resembles myocarditis if the inflammation is centered on the pericardium and subepicardial layer of the myocardium (**Fig. 9**). There is global myocardial dysfunction with frequent right ventricular involvement.[22]

Hypertrophic Cardiomyopathy

Hypertrophic cardiomyopathy, also known as asymmetric septal hypertrophy, is an increasingly recognized disorder, owing partly to the recognition of the breadth of its phenotype.

The disproportionate thickening of the subaortic septum leads to planimetric narrowing of the left ventricular outflow tract (LVOT) during systole (**Fig. 10**). LVOT narrowing increases the velocity of the flow jet, which creates a pressure drop

(Venturi effect). The Venturi effect in turn pulls the anterior leaflet of the mitral valve. The systolic anterior motion of the anterior leaflet of the mitral valve (SAM) further narrows the LVOT, exacerbating the cycle and predisposing to sudden death.[23] SAM is readily detected on cine MR imaging. In addition, the success of targeted ablation of the thickened myocardium in the subaortic septum can be quantified on CMR by observing for the presence or absence of SAM and by measuring the gradient through the LVOT using phase velocity imaging.

LGE, though not a diagnostic criteria for HOCM, does offer prognostic information. Survival is inversely related to the planimetric quantity of LGE. Therefore the presence or absence of LGE can be used in decision making for prophylactic ICDs. The rarer apical form of HOCM lies within

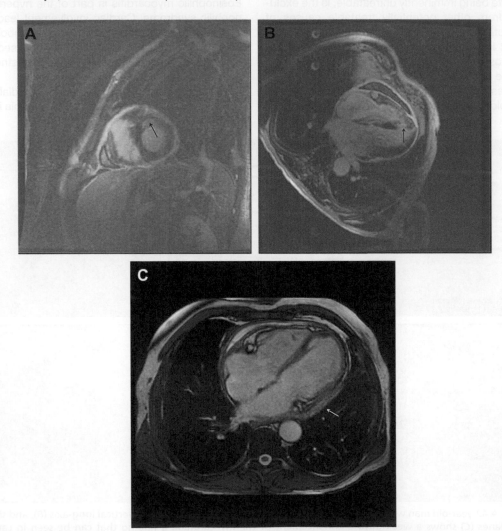

Fig. 9. A 35-year-old man with chest pain, fever, and elevated eosinophils. Scar imaging in the short-axis and 4-chamber planes shows multifocal LGE, which is midmyocardial in location (*arrow* in *A, B*). In addition, there is a pericardial effusion (*arrow* in *C*).

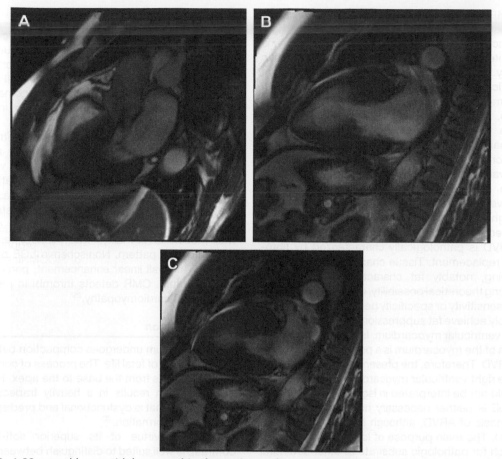

Fig. 10. A 28-year-old man with hypertrophic obstructive cardiomyopathy. Still frame of cine loop in end systole from 3-chamber view of the heart shows asymmetric thickening of the subaortic septum and flow acceleration through the LV outflow tract (A). Still frames of a cine loop in end diastole (B) and end systole (C) in the vertical long-axis view shows thickened basal myocardium and a hyperdynamic LV function.

the acoustic blind spot of echocardiography, owing to the near field effect. CMR readily diagnoses this variant (Fig. 11).[24]

Arrhythmogenic Right Ventricular Dysplasia

Arrhythmogenic right ventricular dysplasia (ARVD) is a cardiomyopathy characterized by fibrous and fatty replacement of the right ventricular myocardium. The disorder may have a familial base.[25] ARVD presents with ventricular tachyarrhythmias, and is a cardiac cause of sudden death in youth. The diagnosis is important because the management includes placement of a prophylactic ICD. A task force has established major and minor criteria for the diagnosis of ARVD.[26] CMR plays an adjunctive role in the diagnosis and a major role in the differential diagnosis, notably in the search for other structural causes of tachyarrhythmias.

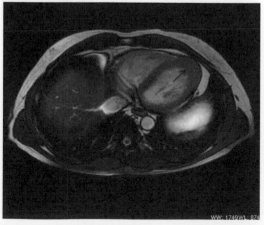

Fig. 11. Still frame of a cine loop in end diastole in the axial plane shows a thickened LV apex, a characteristic finding in the rare apical variant of hypertrophic cardiomyopathy.

CMR enjoys unchallenged superiority in correctly assessing the function of the right ventricle which, owing to its complex geometry, is not interrogated by echo with the same diagnostic clarity. Findings of ARVD on CMR include right ventricular dilation and wall motion abnormalities. Wall motion abnormalities include hypokinesis, akinesis, and dyskinesis, and are particularly suspicious if severe, segmental, or regional, with normal left ventricular function. Wall thinning leads to microaneurysms and macroaneurysms (**Fig. 12**). Outward bulging of the right ventricular free wall is more concerning in diastole.[27] Left ventricle involvement is a late phenomenon, and the degree of right ventricular dysfunction almost invariably exceeds that of the left ventricle.

ARVD is pathologically characterized by fibrofatty replacement. Tissue characterization by MR imaging, notably fat characterization, although a strong theoretical possibility, does not enjoy a reliable sensitivity or specificity because it is difficult to reliably achieve fat suppression of the normally thin right ventricular myocardium. In addition, fat deposition of the myocardium is a process independent of ARVD. Therefore, the presence or absence of fat in the right ventricular myocardium is a finding that should not be interpreted in isolation.[28]

LGE is neither necessary nor sufficient for the diagnosis of ARVD, although it can be present in ARVD. The main purpose of looking for LGE is to search for pathologic substrate of other structural causes of tachyarrhythmias in the right and left ventricles.

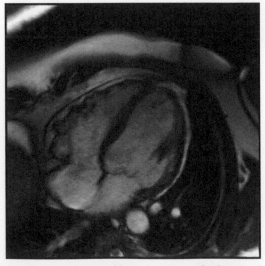

Fig. 12. An 18-year-old man with arrhythmogenic right ventricular dysplasia. Still frame of an axial cine loop shows multiple aneurysms of the right ventricular free wall.

Dilated Cardiomyopathy

Dilated cardiomyopathy is a morphologic descriptor in which there is myocardial dysfunction coupled with dilated heart. There is often compensatory myocardial hypertrophy, but the wall thickness is seldom sufficient to overcome the increased stress due to chamber dilation, incumbent on Laplace's law.

CMR is useful in elucidating the cause in such patients, about one-third of whom have undetected chronic CAD. Another third have a variety of disorders such as myocarditis culminating in this common end point. In one-third a cause is not known (see **Fig. 5**). Findings suggestive of CAD include segmental as opposed to global wall motion abnormality, wall thinning, and an ischemic LGE pattern. Nonischemic LGE pattern includes midwall linear enhancement, particularly in the septum. CMR detects thrombi in patients with dilated cardiomyopathy.[29]

Noncompaction

The myocardium undergoes compaction between 5 and 8 weeks of fetal life. The process of compaction progresses from the base to the apex. Failure of compaction results in a heavily trabeculated myocardium that is dysfunctional and predisposes to thrombus formation.[30]

CMR, by virtue of its superior soft-tissue contrast, is well suited to distinguish between noncompacted and compacted myocardium (**Fig. 13**). In the region of hypertrabeculation there are deep intratrabecular recesses with continuity between the ventricular cavity and the recesses. The ratio of the thickness of the noncompacted myocardium to the compactum is greater than 2.2 in diastole. Noncompaction typically involves the apical and midventricular segments, affecting the lateral and inferior walls. Areas of noncompacted myocardium can have fibrosis, leading to LGE.[31]

Drug-Induced Cardiomyopathy

CMR has a potential role in the follow-up of patients on cardiotoxic chemotherapy, such as anthracyclines, by serial monitoring of the ejection fraction, although this task is more often done by radionuclide ventriculography. However, myocardial damage can be detected by CMR. The LGE pattern described is subepicardial involvement of the inferior and lateral walls.[32]

Autoimmune Diseases

Carditis is a manifestation of autoimmune disease such as systemic lupus erythematosus (SLE). Although no CMR finding is specific for myocardial

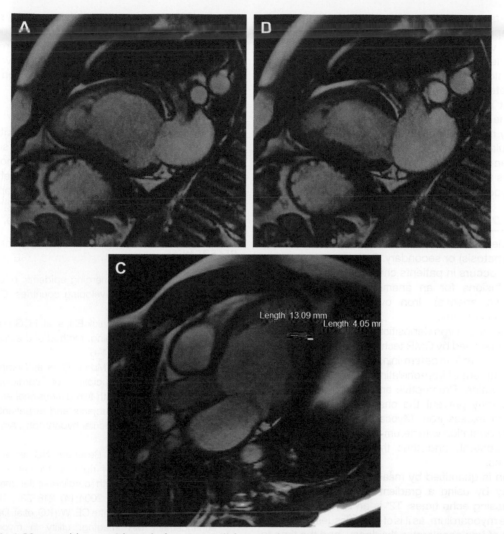

Fig. 13. A 38-year-old man with LV dysfunction. Still frames of a cine loop in end diastole (*A*) and end systole (*B*) show a dilated and severely hypokinetic left ventricle with apical hypertrabeculation. The ratio of the thickness of the noncompacted layer to the compactum in end diastole is greater than 2.2 (*C*). A diagnosis of noncompaction cardiomyopathy was established.

involvement, the presence of LGE in the subepicardial location has been described, and can confirm a high index of suspicion. SLE leads to a verrucous endocarditis (Libman-Sacks endocarditis). The myocardial T1 is higher in patients with active SLE.[33]

Chagas Disease

Chagas disease can affect the heart. The causative agent is *Trypanasoma cruzi*. This entity is endemic in South America. Cardiac involvement is typically seen in the chronic phase in which there is refractory heart failure and tachyarrhythmias. Scar formation is typically midmyocardial and subepicardial, with a predilection for the inferolateral wall of the base.[34]

Metabolic Storage Diseases

Inborn errors of metabolism leading to abnormal accumulation and deposition of certain lipids and polysaccharides can involve the heart. Such disorders can lead to wall thickening, valve thickening, and myocardial dysfunction. One such entity, Anderson-Fabry disease (X-linked disorder of sphingolipid metabolism), is known to mimic hypertrophic cardiomyopathy. The pattern of LGE described is midmyocardial, in the basal free wall of the left ventricle.[35]

Takotsubo Cardiomyopathy

Reversible apical cardiac dysfunction without LGE is the hallmark of takotsubo cardiomyopathy.

Tako-tsubo, Japanese for octopus fishing pot, is the appearance likened to this condition on left-sided ventriculography.[36]

Patients present with chest pain, ST-segment elevation, and no offending coronary lesions on catheter angiography. The precipitating event might be an acutely emotional event. The apical segments of the heart are akinetic/dyskinetic. Many mechanisms for this dysfunction have been postulated; the suggested common pathway is an ischemic insult (either large vessel or small vessel) that is followed by reperfusion. The technical term is myocardial stunning.

Iron Deposition in the Heart

Iron deposition in the heart may be primary (hemochromatosis) or secondary. Secondary iron deposition occurs in patients chronically dependent on transfusions for an anemic state (thalassemia, aplastic anemia). Iron overload may lead to cardiomyopathy.

Myocardial iron deposition can be both detected and quantified by CMR techniques. The quantification is valuable in determining the need and success of treatment of iron-chelating agents such as desferioxamine. Preemptive and/or aggressive treatment may prevent the onset of cardiomyopathy due to excess iron. Myocardial iron content has poor correlation with serum iron parameters or liver iron content, and thus these cannot serve as proxies.

Iron is quantified by measuring the T2 star (T2*) decay by using a gradient echo sequence with increasing echo times. T2* is an inherent property of the myocardium, as it is of other tissues. The presence of iron accelerates the decay, and the time to decay is inversely proportional to the myocardial iron content. Decay times of less than 20 milliseconds indicate myocardial iron overload.[37]

Valvular Heart Disease

Whereas echocardiography is the preferred modality for the assessment of valvular heart disease, CMR can provide both anatomic and functional evaluation of the valves. Phase velocity imaging provides information about forward and reverse flows through the valve orifice, thereby quantifying regurgitant fractions. Peak velocity through the modified Bernoulli equation can quantify the gradient through the valve.[38]

Even if CMR is not considered the first-line modality for suspected valvular heart disease, its ability to provide this information is important, as it allows a comprehensive cardiac assessment. The breadth of information provided by CMR technically allows the possibility of obtaining all the requisite information in a single study (a one-stop shop). Equally important, in a patient with multiple coexisting cardiac pathologies CMR can give the relative contributions of ischemic, nonischemic, and valvular dysfunction to the overall cardiac dysfunction.

SUMMARY

CMR's excellent soft-tissue contrast with its detection and spatial characterization of scar is the single most important reason why this modality is invaluable in making the distinction between ischemic and nonischemic cardiomyopathy. CMR occupies a leading role in the diagnostic and clinical decision making in heart failure.

REFERENCES

1. Reddy KS, Yusuf S. Emerging epidemic of cardiovascular disease in developing countries. Circulation 1998;97:596–601.
2. Lanzer P, Barta C, Botvinick EH, et al. ECG-synchronized cardiac MR imaging: method and evaluation. Radiology 1985;155:681–6.
3. Grothues F, Smith GC, Moon JC, et al. Comparison of interstudy reproducibility of cardiovascular magnetic resonance with two-dimensional echocardiography in normal subjects and in patients with heart failure or left ventricular hypertrophy. Am J Cardiol 2002;90:29–34.
4. Grothues F, Moon JC, Bellenger NG, et al. Interstudy reproducibility of right ventricular volumes, function, and mass with cardiovascular magnetic resonance. Am Heart J 2004;147:218–23.
5. Vogel-Claussen J, Rochitte CE, Wu KC, et al. Delayed enhancement MR imaging: utility in myocardial assessment. Radiographics 2006;26(3):795–810.
6. McCrohon JA, Moon JC, Prasad SK, et al. Differentiation of heart failure related to dilated cardiomyopathy and coronary artery disease using gadolinium-enhanced cardiovascular magnetic resonance. Circulation 2003;108:54–9.
7. Fleckenstein JL, Archer BT, Barker BA, et al. Fast short tau inversion-recovery MR imaging. Radiology 1991;179:499–504.
8. Verhaert D, Thavendiranathan P, Giri S, et al. Direct T2 quantification of myocardial edema in acute ischemic injury. JACC Cardiovasc Imaging 2011; 4(3):269–78.
9. Cummings KW, Bhalla S, Javidan-Nejad C, et al. A pattern-based approach to assessment of delayed enhancement in nonischemic cardiomyopathy at MR imaging. Radiographics 2009;29:89–103.
10. Bello D, Fieno D, Kim RJ, et al. Infarct morphology identifies patients with substrate for sustained ventricular tachycardia. J Am Coll Cardiol 2005;45: 1104–8.

11. Nazarian S, Bluemke DA, Lardo AC, et al. Magnetic resonance assessment of the substrate for inducible ventricular tachycardia in nonischemic cardiomyopathy. Circulation 2005;112:2821–5.

12. Lehrke S, Lossnitzer D, Schöb M, et al. Use of cardiovascular magnetic resonance for risk stratification in chronic heart failure: prognostic value of late gadolinium enhancement in patients with nonischaemic dilated cardiomyopathy. Heart 2011;97:727–32.

13. Moon JC, McKenna WJ, McCrohon JA, et al. Toward clinical risk assessment in hypertrophic cardiomyopathy with gadolinium cardiovascular magnetic resonance. J Am Coll Cardiol 2003;41(9):1561–7.

14. Bleeker GB, Kaandorp TA, Lamb HJ, et al. Effect of posterolateral scar tissue on clinical and echocardiographic improvement after cardiac resynchronization therapy. Circulation 2006;113:969–76.

15. Iles L, Pfluger H, Lefkovits L, et al. Myocardial fibrosis predicts appropriate device therapy in patients with implantable cardioverter-defibrillators for primary prevention of sudden cardiac death. J Am Coll Cardiol 2011;57:821–8.

16. Borchert B, Lawrenz T, Bartelsmeier M, et al. Utility of endomyocardial biopsy guided by delayed enhancement areas on magnetic resonance imaging in the diagnosis of cardiac sarcoidosis. Clin Res Cardiol 2007;96(10):759–62.

17. Mahrholdt H, Goedecke C, Wagner A. Cardiovascular magnetic resonance assessment of human myocarditis: a comparison to histology and molecular pathology. Circulation 2004;109(10):1250–8.

18. Matsui Y, Iwai K, Tachibana T, et al. Clinicopathological study of fatal myocardial sarcoidosis. Ann N Y Acad Sci 1976;278:455–69.

19. Vignaux O. Cardiac sarcoidosis: spectrum of MRI features. AJR Am J Roentgenol 2005;184(1):249–54.

20. Falk RH, Rubinow A, Cohen AS. Cardiac arrhythmias in systemic amyloidosis: correlation with echocardiographic abnormalities. J Am Coll Cardiol 1984;3:107–13.

21. Maceira AM, Joshi J, Prasad SK, et al. Cardiovascular magnetic resonance in cardiac amyloidosis. Circulation 2005;111:186–93.

22. Ogbogu PU, Rosing DR, Horne MK 3rd. Cardiovascular manifestations of hypereosinophilic syndromes. Immunol Allergy Clin North Am 2007;27(3):457–75.

23. Maron BJ. Hypertrophic cardiomyopathy: a systematic review. JAMA 2002;287(10):1308–20.

24. Chun EJ, Choi SI, Jin KN, et al. Hypertrophic cardiomyopathy: assessment with MR imaging and multidetector CT. Radiographics 2010;30:1309–28. DOI: 10.1148/rg.305095074.

25. Thiene G, Nava A, Corrado D, et al. Right ventricular cardiomyopathy and sudden death in young people. N Engl J Med 1988;318:129–33.

26. Marcus FI, McKenna WJ, Sherrill D, et al. Diagnosis of arrhythmogenic right ventricular cardiomyopathy/dysplasia. proposed modification of the task force criteria. Circulation 2010;121:1533–41.

27. Kayser HW, van der Wall EE, Sivananthan MU, et al. Diagnosis of arrhythmogenic right ventricular dysplasia: a review. Radiographics 2002;22:639–50.

28. Burke AP, Farb A, Tashko G, et al. Arrhythmogenic right ventricular cardiomyopathy and fatty replacement of the right ventricular myocardium: are they different disease? Circulation 1998;97:1571–80.

29. Assomull RG, Prasad SK, Lynne J, et al. Cardiovascular magnetic resonance, fibrosis, and prognosis in dilated cardiomyopathy. J Am Coll Cardiol 2006;48:1977–85.

30. Weiford BC, Subbarao VD, Mulhern KM. Noncompaction of the ventricular myocardium. Circulation 2004;109(24):2965–71.

31. Jassal DS, Nomura CH, Neilan TG, et al. Delayed enhancement cardiac MR imaging in noncompaction of left ventricular myocardium. J Cardiovasc Magn Reson 2006;8(3):489–91.

32. Wassmuth R, Hauser IA, Schuler K, et al. Subclinical cardiotoxic effects of anthracyclines as assessed by magnetic resonance imaging—a pilot study. Am Heart J 2001;141(6):1007–13.

33. Abdel-Aty H, Siegle N, Natusch A, et al. Myocardial tissue characterization in systemic lupus erythematosus: value of a comprehensive cardiovascular magnetic resonance approach. Lupus 2008;17:561–7.

34. Bocchi EA, Kalil R, Bacal F, et al. Magnetic resonance imaging in chronic Chagas' disease: correlation with endomyocardial biopsy findings and gallium-67 cardiac uptake. Echocardiography 1998;15:279–88.

35. Moon JC, Sachdev B, Elkington AG, et al. Gadolinium enhanced cardiovascular magnetic resonance in Anderson-Fabry disease: evidence for a disease specific abnormality of the myocardial interstitium. Eur Heart J 2003;24:2151–5.

36. Akashi YJ, Goldstein DS, Barbaro G, et al. Takotsubo cardiomyopathy: a new form of acute, reversible heart failure. Circulation 2008;118:2754–62.

37. Anderson LJ, Holden S, Davis B, et al. Cardiovascular T2-star (T2*) magnetic resonance for the early diagnosis of myocardial iron overload. Eur Heart J 2001;22:2171–9.

38. Glockner JF, Johnston DL, McGee KP. Evaluation of cardiac valvular disease with MR imaging: qualitative and quantitative techniques. Radiographics 2003;23:e9.

MR Imaging of Myocardial Scar, with Electrophysiology Applications

Benoit Desjardins, MD, PhD

KEYWORDS

- Myocardial scar
- Magnetic resonance imaging
- Cardiac electrophysiology

Cardiac arrhythmia affect more than 14 million people in the United States and is responsible for more than 800,000 annual hospital visits and half a million deaths per year.[1] Some arrhythmias are immediately life threatening (eg, ventricular tachyarrhythmia secondary to myocardial infarct), whereas other arrhythmias are not immediately life threatening but are responsible for important morbidity, such as strokes (eg, atrial fibrillation).

Fifty percent of cases of sudden cardiac death (SCD) occur in subjects with a prior history of myocardial disease.[2] To prevent potentially fatal arrhythmia, more than 300,000 subjects per year with known heart disease receive implantable cardioverter-defibrillators (ICDs). Current clinical guidelines for risk stratification to determine who needs an ICD depend on cardiac function: subjects with preserved left ventricular (LV) function do not require ICDs, whereas subjects with depressed LV function most likely benefit from ICDs.[1,3,4] There has been a reduction in mortality in subjects with

depressed LV function who have received an ICD, but depressed cardiac function is only a surrogate marker for arrhythmia. The etiology of most arrhythmia is a combination of abnormal myocardial substrate (scar) combined with transient electrophysiologic events.[5] So direct assessment of the arrhythmogenic substrate and electrophysiologic assessment of the heart might prove useful for risk stratification.

Myocardial scar acts as an arrhythmogenic substrate: subjects with increasing amount of scars show increasing arrhythmia, increasing cardiac failure, and increasing mortality.[6] Small scars can be highly arrhythmogenic, without significantly depressing the LV function, so these subjects are typically not candidates for ICDs but really need one. Only a small percentage of subjects who experience SCD have an ICD.[4] Alternatively, some diseases depress LV function but have no scar and no significant increase in risk of arrhythmia, yet these subjects can receive an ICD using current

The author has nothing to disclose.
The use of Gadolinium for Cardiac MRI is not an FDA approved indication.
Department of Radiology, University of Pennsylvania, 3400 Spruce Street, Philadelphia, PA 19104, USA
E-mail address: bdmdphd@me.com

PET Clin 6 (2011) 489–502
doi:10.1016/j.cpet.2011.10.004

risk stratification criteria. Only 5% of subjects who receive an ICD actually trigger the device for shocks every year.[4] There is, therefore, a discrepancy between subjects who receive an ICD and subjects who really need one. Because ICDs are expensive devices, there is need for better clinical guidelines for risk stratification, and direct imaging of the arrhythmogenic substrate seems promising for this purpose.

Electrophysiologic assessment of the heart for risk stratification purposes could also prove useful, independently or in combination with substrate imaging. Many electrophysiologic techniques have been investigated, such as T-wave alternans, QT dispersion, heart rate variability, ventricular ectopy, and nonsustained ventricular tachycardia, but these techniques have low sensitivity.[1] These techniques are not discussed in this article.

The purpose of this article is to review the increasing role of cardiac MR imaging to quantitatively assess myocardial scar in the context of clinical cardiac electrophysiology. After a quick overview of the biologic aspects of myocardial scar, two imaging techniques currently used to routinely image scar in cardiac electrophysiology (EP) contexts are described, MR imaging and electroanatomic mapping (EAM), and their relationship is explained. The main clinical issues involving MR imaging for cardiac EP are then reviewed, including imaging in cardiomyopathy (both ischemic and nonischemic), imaging for cardiac ablation therapy, and imaging of subjects with intracardiac devices.

IMAGING OF MYOCARDIAL SCAR IN ELECTROPHYSIOLOGY

Multiple imaging modalities are useful for clinical EP. Fluoroscopy (**Fig. 1**A) depicts the position of EP catheters as well as cardiac chamber anatomy after injection of intravenous (IV) contrast agent. It has been used to guide most EP procedures for many years. Transthoracic or intracardiac ultrasound (see **Fig. 1**B) dynamically depicts anatomy along specific imaging planes and is becoming increasing useful in EP. CT (**Fig. 2**A, B) and MR imaging (see **Fig. 2**C) provide full 3-D imaging of anatomy and function and are providing 3-D mapping information for EP procedures. As in many other areas of cardiology, there has been a move in imaging in EP away from depicting purely anatomic information to depicting quantitative physiologic information, such as function, perfusion, flow, and scar characterization.

Myocardial Scar and IV Contrast Agents

Myocardial scar in both acute and chronic myocardial infarct can be imaged by different modalities using IV contrast agents. Two elements help distinguish scar from normal myocardium: the volumes of distribution and the kinetics of distribution of the IV contrast agents. First, these extracellular contrast agents have low molecular weight and distribute in the interstitium of the myocardium. In acute infarct, there is disruption of the cellular membranes, leading to access by the IV contrast agent to the intracellular

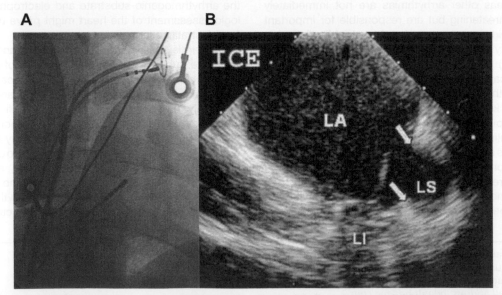

Fig. 1. Two imaging modalities often used in cardiac EP are (*A*) fluoroscopy and (*B*) intracardiac echo. ICE, intracardiac echocardiography; LA, left atrium; LI, left inferior pulmonary vein; LS, left superior pulmonary vein.

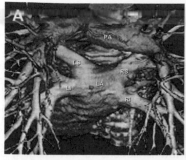
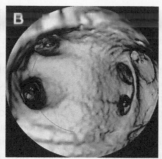
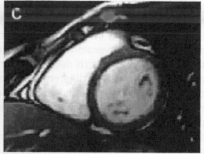

Fig. 2. Volumetric imaging modalities, such as CT and MR imaging, provide detailed 3-D and dynamic information about the heart. (*A*) Surface shaded view of the posterior aspect of the heart showing the left atrium and PVs. (*B*) Endocardial surface shaded view of the left atrium showing the ostia of the PVs. (*C*) Single short-axis SSFP MR image, which is part of a dynamic sequence to characterize cardiac function.

compartment by diffusion as well as increase of the size of the interstitium due to local edema.[7,8] In chronic infarct, there is enlargement of the interstitium with decrease in number of cells and increase in collagen content. Thus, in both acute and chronic infarct, there is increase of the volume of distribution of the IV contrast agent in scar compared with normal myocardium. Second, there is delay in the washout of the contrast agent from the scar compared with the normal myocardium, so when delayed imaging is performed, there is a greater concentration of contrast agent in the scar compared with the normal myocardium.[9]

The center (core) of the infarct typically contains solid scar. The periphery of the infarct (border zone) contains intermeshing of normal myocardial cells and fibrosis. This intermeshing modifies both the local electrophysiologic properties and the geometry of the local myocardium. The scar border zone seems to play an important role in the disruption of electrical conduction and the generation of reentrant circuits in the myocardium.

If scar is imaged in the first week after infarction, the presence of microvascular obstruction in some subjects due to microemboli combined with edema can prevent the IV contrast from reaching the central portions of the scar.[10] The IV contrast, therefore, fails to concentrate within the core of the scar but concentrates in the periphery of the scar.

During the first month after infarct, there is healing of the infarct and cardiac remodeling.[11,12] There is decrease in the edema within and around the infarct. There is local inflammation resulting in the resorption of the necrotic tissue as well as local deposition of collagen. This results in decrease in the area of accumulation of the IV contrast agent. This is accompanied by chamber dilatation and compensatory hypertrophy of the surrounding myocardium.

Scar Imaging by Magnetic Resonance

The most commonly used technique to detect myocardial scar by MR imaging is a technique of delayed enhancement (DE)-MR imaging using gadolinium-based contrast agents (**Fig. 3**).[13,14] The contrast agent creates T1 shortening, increasing signal on MR imaging. A dose of 0.1 to 0.2 mmol/kg of contrast agent is injected IV. T1-weighted MR imaging is typically performed from 10 to 30 minutes after the administration of the IV contrast agent.[15] To improve the difference in signal between the normal myocardium and the scar, an inversion recovery pulse is used to null the signal of the normal myocardium. On the resulting DE-MR images, the normal myocardium is very dark and the scar is very bright, typically at least 5

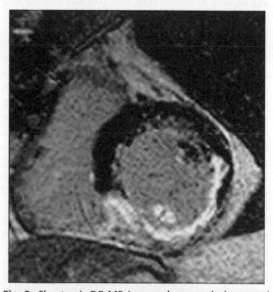

Fig. 3. Short-axis DE-MR image shows a dark normal myocardium, due to good nulling, with a partly subendocardial and partly transmural scar showing as bright signal.

times brighter than the normal myocardium. The inversion time represents the time between the application of the inversion pulse and the image acquisition. The inversion time of the pulse required to null the myocardium is determined empirically by acquiring images with different inversion times and determining on which images the normal myocardium has the lowest signal.[16] 2-D imaging can be performed, where a stack of 10 to 14 parallel images is acquired along the short axis of the LV as well as orthogonal long axis images to decrease the possibility of artifacts being interpreted as infarcts. In-plane resolution is approximately 1 to 2 mm and slice thickness 8 to 10 mm with one breath hold per image. 2-D phase-sensitive inversion recovery sequences can also be performed, which can null the myocardium over a wider range of inversion times.[17] 3-D imaging is also available with decreased slice thickness and a total of 1 to 2 breath holds but worse nulling of the normal myocardium. 3-D whole-heart imaging can also be performed with free breathing, electrocardiogram (ECG) gating, and navigator gating, to produce 1-mm isotropic resolution images with excellent nulling of the normal myocardium.[18]

On DE-MR images, the MR signal at the core of the infarct is typically higher than the signal at the border zone. Microvascular obstruction, however, shows as very low signal surrounded by high signal. The size of the area of microvascular obstruction is significant prognostically.[19] Both chronic and acute infarct show up as bright signal on DE- MR images, but T2-weighed imaging shows bright signal only in acute scar due to local edema and can be used to discriminate between acute and chronic scar.[20]

Quantification of myocardial scar can be performed manually or semiautomatically.[21] The size and degree of transmurality of scar are typically quantified. To assess absolute size, the scar can either be traced manually or segmented using a thresholding approach. Manual tracing is time consuming and user dependent and can show significant intraobserver and interobserver variability. A more automatic approach using a threshold of signal intensity is preferred. Unlike CT, where values of attenuation are normalized and constant from examination to examination, the intensity values of pixels on MR images are sequence dependent and their absolute value is meaningless clinically. Thresholding is, therefore, always performed relative to the normal myocardium. Although there is still no consensus as to which thresholding techniques are best, comparison with infarct sizes as determined by triphenyl-tetrozolium chloride staining of ex vivo hearts[22,23] shows that a threshold of 2 SDs from normal can

be used to adequately segment scar.[23] Thresholding with a technique of full width at half maximum might be even more accurate to segment scar.[21] In addition to thresholding of scar, the appropriate delineation of the endocardial and epicardial contours is required to assess scar as percentage of the entire myocardial mass and to assess transmural extent of scar. Both manual and semiautomatic techniques have been proposed to identify the endocardial and epicardial contours.

There are a few limitations to MR imaging of scar. In subjects with renal failure, the administration of gadolinium-based IV contrast agents is contraindicated due to the risk of nephrogenic systemic sclerosis.[24] T1-weighted–based imaging techniques are being developed to image scar without the need for IV contrast agents.[25] The administration of IV MR contrast agent is also contraindicated in subjects who are pregnant, given the potential risks to the fetus. Some subjects who are claustrophobic, are too fat, or have some metallic implants are not good candidates for MR imaging. Although the presence of pacemaker or implanted cardiac defibrillators used to be a contraindication, MR imaging of the heart and other parts of the body can now safely be performed with proper supervision in these subjects. Most techniques of cardiac MR imaging require ECG gating to produce both static and dynamic images of the heart. In subjects with severe arrhythmia, ECG gating cannot be used. Real-time imaging can be performed in such subjects to produce dynamic images, although DE images typically are blurry. Most cardiac MR imaging requires breath holding. Navigator-gated imaging, which tracks the position of the diaphragm, can be used for free-breathing imaging in subjects who cannot hold their breath or for long imaging sequences.

Scar Imaging by Electroanatomic Mapping

The main imaging technique for electrophysiologic assessment of the heart is EAM, often used in the course of radiofrequency (RF) cardiac ablation therapy of arrhythmia.[26] For endocardial mapping, a femoral approach is used to advance a catheter all the way to the heart, using a direct venous path to access the right ventricle or a retrograde aortic path to access the LV. Near the tip of the catheter is a series of recording electrodes, which can directly measure voltage at the surface of the myocardium. For epicardial mapping, a transpericardial approach is used to measure voltages at the epicardial surface of the heart. An approach via the coronary veins can offer limited epicardial mapping. The electrodes on the catheter can measure bipolar voltages and unipolar voltages as well infer timing information in the cardiac depolarization. A 3-D mapping system (eg, CARTO XP, Biosense Webster, Diamond Bar, California) records the position of the tip of the catheter in 3-D space when measurements are performed. A cardiac voltage surface map is generated from 200 to 300 endocardial or epicardial measurements during sinus rhythm, each localized in 3-D space by the mapping system (**Fig. 4**). On the electroanatomic map, low voltage measurements are illustrated in red and normal voltage measurements in purple. Scar tissue has low voltage measurements (<1.5 mV bipolar), so areas in red color correspond to areas of scar. Additional catheters are advanced into the heart for the purpose of programmed stimulations to try to induce arrhythmia during EP procedures, and other catheters are used for RF ablation therapy. Such imaging studies are the current basis for the detailed electroanatomic assessment of the heart. They are used to identify scar, identify critical sites for arrhythmia, and ablate those sites.

There is excellent correspondence between the scar distribution as determined by EAM and the scar distribution on DE-MR imaging.[27] The critical sites for arrhythmia are typically located within or at the periphery of the scar, and are the targets for ablation therapy. The pattern of scar on MR imaging can predict success of ablation. A recent study showed that in subjects with inducible ventricular tachycardia, all the critical sites for arrhythmia were located in scar[27]—55% of the critical sites were associated with endocardial scar on MR imaging; 70% of those sites were successfully ablated from an endocardial approach, and 30% had an intramural component and only partial success at ablation using an endocardial approach; 15% of the critical sites were associated with an epicardial scar on MR imaging and all of them were successfully ablated via an epicardial approach; and 30% of the critical sites were associated with an intramural scar on MR imaging, and their ablation was ineffective.

There are some limitations to EAM. First, poor contact of the catheter with the myocardial surface results in low measured voltages, which can mimic scar. On the endocardial surface, this can be due to the presence of trabeculations or thrombus in the cardiac chamber. On the epicardial surface, this can be due to thick epicardial fat separating the myocardium from the catheter tip in the pericardial space (**Fig. 5**).[28] Second, there is limited sampling during EAM. The surface map is a computer interpolation of the measurement points, but poorly sampled areas of the myocardium lack data to properly characterize the extent of scar (**Fig. 6**). Third, subendocardial or subepicardial scars produce low voltages on the respective endocardial and epicardial maps, but intramural scar might be difficult to detect from either an endocardial or epicardial approach. Unipolar voltages rather than bipolar voltages are proving useful to identify scar located deeper in the wall of the myocardium.[27]

CLINICAL ISSUES
Cardiomyopathy

Ischemic cardiomyopathy
After a myocardial infarct, subjects have increased risk for ventricular tachyarrhythmia, which can lead to SCD. The arrhythmia can be of early onset (<48 h) after the infarct, which is typically an epiphenomenon of the myocardial infarct, or late onset, where the scar acts as arrhythmogenic substrate; 25% of the arrhythmic death occurs within the first 3 months after an infarct, and 50% occur within the first year after an infarct.

Imaging plays an important role in ischemic cardiomyopathy. General anatomic imaging and functional imaging can assess the development of heart failure and cardiac remodeling and is used for risk stratification for ICD placement. Subjects with preserved LV function (>40%) do not require an ICD; subjects with depressed function (<35%) likely require an ICD; and subjects in the 35% to 40% range are closely followed up.[4]

Imaging can assess the degree of atherosclerotic disease in the coronary arteries and the resulting first-pass perfusion abnormalities in the

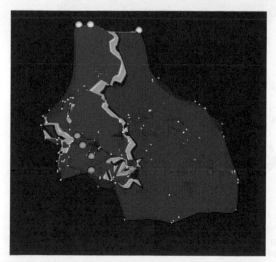

Fig. 4. 3-D electroanatomic map of the endocardial surface of the LV. The red area represents a large posterior and inferior scar, whereas the purple area represents normal myocardium.

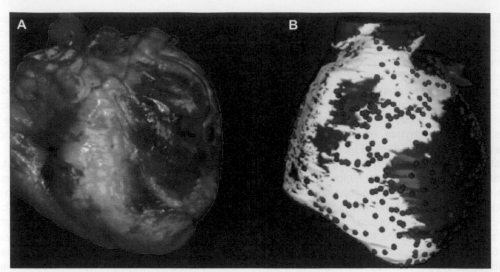

Fig. 5. The effect of epicardial fat on the epicardial electroanatomic map. (*A*) Gross pathology of an explanted heart, showing significant epicardial fat along the AV groove (*B*) 3-D map of fat extracted from CT data, superposed on the individual epicardial measurement points, reveal that the low voltages (*red*) are due to significant epicardial fat attenuating the epicardial measurements.

myocardium. Scar imaging can assess the size and degree of transmurality of scar, to determine if revascularization can be useful (**Fig. 7**).

The scar on DE-MR imaging in ischemic cardiomyopathy is always located in a vascular distribution territory. There is always a subendocardial component and variable transmural extent. Chronic scar is accompanied by thinning of the myocardium and associated wall motion abnormality, cardiac remodeling, and sometimes

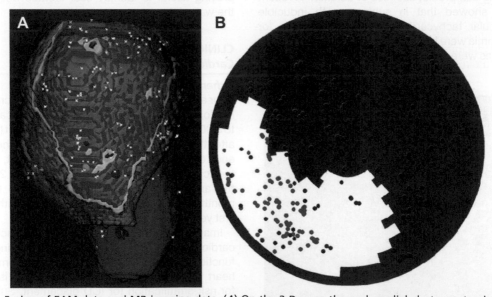

Fig. 6. Fusion of EAM data and MR imaging data. (*A*) On the 3-D map, the endocardial electroanatomic map is projected on the segmented endocardial surface as determined by MR imaging. The scar by EAM is in red, and the scar by MR imaging is in gray. There is only partial overlap of the scar as assessed by the two modalities. (*B*) The same data represented as a polar projection map of the DE-MR imaging, with scar in white and normal myocardium in black, superimposed to the individual measurement points on the EAM (*red*, low voltage; *blue*, normal voltage). Again there is partial match at the level of the scar, but this view demonstrates insufficient sampling of the scar by EAM, leading to underestimation of the extent of the scar on the 3-D electroanatomic map illustrated in (*A*).

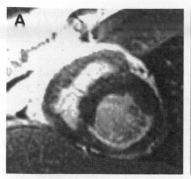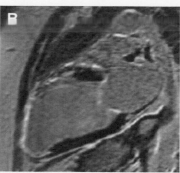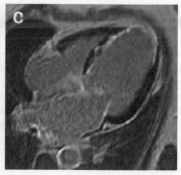

Fig. 7. DE-MR imaging showing bright scar on a background of normal darker myocardium. (*A*) Short-axis image of the LV shows subendocardial scar in the inferoseptal and inferolateral walls. (*B*) Two-chamber long-axis of the LV in a different subject shows transmural extent of scar in the anterior wall and apex. (*C*) Four-chamber long-axis view of the LV shows transmural apical scar and subendocardial septal scar.

calcifications and fatty involution. Imaging can also detect complications of myocardial infarct, which have a prognostic value. Such complications include mitral regurgitation, ventricular septal defect, thrombus, LV aneurysm and pseudoaneurysm, and pericardial effusion (**Fig. 8**).

Both the size of the total infarct and the size of the border zone correlate with inducibility of arrhythmia on EP studies.[29,30] Heterogeneity of scar in the myocardial wall and even in the papillary muscles has been related to inducibility of arrhythmia.[31] Scar distribution involving 25% to 75% of wall thickness is predictive of inducible VT.[32] The amount of border zone is predictive of ventricular arrhythmia post-ICD, can distinguish subjects with inducible versus noninducible ventricular tachycardia,[30] and can predict survival.[29]

Nonischemic cardiomyopathy

Scar and areas of fibrosis are also seen in nonischemic cardiomyopathy.[33,34] They act as an arrhythmogenic substrate and can be imaged by DE-MR imaging. Surviving muscle bundles within scar are likely responsible for arrhythmia.[35]

The patterns of fibrosis in nonischemic cardiomyopathy are more varied than in ischemic cardiomyopathy and do not follow typical coronary artery perfusion territories.[36] Scar distribution can be subendocardial, transmural, intramural, subepicardial, and at the insertion points of the right ventricle on the LV.[33,37] The presence and amount of scar in nonischemic cardiomyopathy has been associated with the inducibility of arrhythmia,[32] the rate of ICD shocks, future cardiac events, hospitalization, and mortality.[38,39]

Hypertrophic cardiomyopathy (HCM) involves myocardial walls that are greater than 12 mm in thickness. Asymmetric septal hypertrophy is the most common type. The etiology is commonly congenital, but a less frequent cause is Fabry disease. HCM is associated with increased incidence of arrhythmia,[40] syncope, acute myocardial

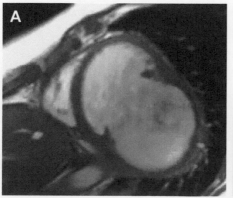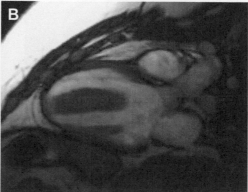

Fig. 8. SSFP images of the heart illustrate two potential complications after infarct. (*A*) There is aneurysmal dilatation of the inferolateral wall after infarct. (*B*) There is a large thrombus filling part of the LV and attached to a thinned infarcted apex.

infarct, exertional angina, and SCD. Imaging in HCM is multifaceted and covers anatomy, function, and scar. For each 1-mm increase in wall thickness, there is a 2-fold to 3-fold increase in arrhythmia. For each 5-mm increase is wall thickness or 50 g/m^2 in cardiac mass, there is a 2-fold increase in SCD. Arrhythmia is more severe when the hypertrophy is asymmetric. Functional imaging can assess functional obstruction of the LV outflow tract in HCM as well as valvular problems, such as systolic anterior motion of the anterior leaflet of the mitral valve, leading to functional subaortic stenosis and functional mitral regurgitation.

Normal cardiac hypertrophy can also occur in athletes as a result of training, and 40% of sudden death in athletes is due to HCM. Imaging can be used to distinguish normal and pathologic hypertrophy in athletes. Pathologic hypertrophy involves wall thickness above 16 mm, is asymmetric, is accompanied by a decrease in size of the LV cavity, an enlarged left atrial size, an impaired LV relaxation, lack of response to deconditioning, and a positive family history.

To predict SCD in HCM, clinical markers are used but are imprecise.[40] Subjects with HCM also have increased fibrosis and scar, as determined at autopsy of HCM subjects with SCD. They have 8 times more fibrosis than normal controls and 3 times more fibrosis than subjects with hypertension.[41] This fibrosis can be imaged by DE-MR imaging and is typically patchy and located in the intramural portion of the hypertrophied walls (**Fig. 9**) and at the insertion point of the right ventricle on the LV.[42] It has been associated with increased incidence of ventricular tachyarrhythmia on Holter monitoring.[43] A rare cause of cardiac hypertrophy is Fabry disease,[34] an enzyme

deficiency. Half of the subjects with Fabry disease show scar on MR imaging,[44] with a pattern predominant in the inferolateral wall with sparing of the subendocardium.

Myocarditis involves focal or multifocal inflammation of the myocardium and can affect young subjects. Subjects with myocarditis are at increased risk of ventricular tachycardia and SCD. The acutely inflamed myocardium and chronic fibrotic sequelae of myocarditis can be imaged by DE-MR imaging.[45,46] The distribution of scar on DE-MR imaging is typically in a subepicardial or intramural location (**Fig. 10**).

Sarcoidosis involves the focal or multifocal deposition of granulomata in the myocardium, leading to chronic scars.[34] These have been found in 50% of sarcoidosis subjects at autopsy and form an arrhythmogenic substrate.[47] Arrhythmia is present in 25% to 50% of subjects with cardiac sarcoidosis and correlates with the degree of severity of sarcoidosis.[47,48] On DE-MR imaging, one or more foci of high signal are found scattered throughout the myocardium, predominantly in the basal lateral portion of the LV (**Fig. 11**).[49,50]

Chagas disease is due to a parasite, which causes diffuse myocardial inflammation, leading to fibrosis and scarring. Subjects are at increased risk of arrhythmia, which correlates with the degree of fibrosis. On DE-MR imaging, there is abnormal signal in a subepicardial distribution, typically at the base of the heart on the lateral wall.[51]

Pulmonary Veins Ablation

Atrial fibrillation (AF) is a disorder where the atria show chaotic electrical activity (350–600 beats per minute) causing quiver instead of an organized contraction. It affects 2.4 million adults in the United States and is expected to affect more

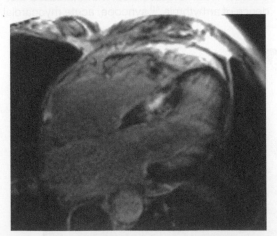

Fig. 9. Four-chamber DE-MR image in HCM illustrates asymmetric thickening of the septum and bright intramural signal in the thickened septum due to fibrosis.

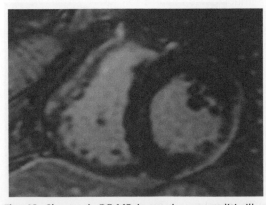

Fig. 10. Short-axis DE-MR image in myocarditis illustrates a large area of subepicardial enhancement in the inferolateral wall.

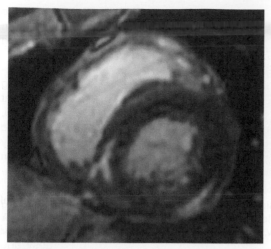

Fig. 11. Short-axis DE-MR image in sarcoidosis shows patchy midmyocardial enhancement in the inferoseptal and inferolateral walls.

than 5 million people by 2040, given that the prevalence increases with age and the population is getting older. Approximately 10% of subjects older than 80 years have atrial fibrillation. It is the most common arrhythmic cause of hospitalization and results in a 2-fold increase in mortality and 5-fold increase in stroke.[52] This is most often caused by excitable tissue extending from the left atrium into the pulmonary veins (PVs). A common therapy is modification of the left atrial substrate by linear ablation around the ostia of the PVs or deeper in the left atrium, resulting in electrical isolation of the PVs. Long-term atrial fibrillation also leads to electrical, contractile, and structural remodeling of the left atrium, leading to persistence of the arrhythmia. The end result of the remodeling process is loss of myocytes and increased fibrosis in the left atrium.[53]

Imaging has multiple roles for cardiac ablation. Before the ablation procedure, imaging is used for anatomic planning purposes, to identify the ostial diameter of the PVs for proper lasso catheter selection, to measure the length to first-order branches, and to identify the existence of additional PVs or of abnormal pulmonary venous return.[54] In addition, imaging is used to measure the shape and volume of the left atrium and to identify any thrombus in the left atrial appendage, which would be a contraindication to an ablation procedure. A dilated left atrium is associated with increase in recurrence of atrial fibrillation[55] and atrial tachycardia[56] postablation.

The esophagus is in close contact to the posterior left atrial wall and may lie within the ablation zone. There is marked variation in the anatomic relationship between esophagus and left atrium, and significant adipose tissue between the esophagus and left atrium can insulate the esophagus from thermal injury during the ablation procedure.[57] Thermal injury to the esophagus during ablation can result in atrial-esophageal fistula, which can be fatal. Other relevant structures can be imaged before the ablation procedure, such as the pulmonary arteries and airways[58] and the right phrenic nerve.[59]

During the ablation, imaging can be used for guidance purposes. The 3-D maps obtained by MR imaging or CT can be imported into specialized systems and fused to the electroanatomic map progressively obtained during the ablation procedure.[60] Image integration was show in some studies to improve the clinical outcome of the ablation procedure and slightly decrease the duration of the procedure and fluoroscopy time.[61]

After the ablation, imaging is used to assess complications to the ablation as well as to assess iatrogenic scar formation in the left atrium or around the ostia of the PVs. The most frequent complication is PV stenosis (up to 42% of cases). Other complications include PV thrombosis, PV dissection, pulmonary infarction, pulmonary hypertension, pleural and pericardial effusions, pericarditis, cardiac perforation, and systemic emboli as well as catheter site hematoma or arteriovenous fistula. Edema in the left atrial wall can be seen in 95% of ostial isolation and 100% of antral isolation. The severity of the edema is related to the amount of RF energy deposited during the procedure and is significantly greater in antral isolation than in ostial isolation. One month after the procedure, the atrial wall edema has resolved.[62]

An RF ablation procedure produces lesions in the myocardium similar to that of a regular scar. After PV ablation, bright signal in the wall of the left atrium around the ostia of the PVs can be seen on DE-MR imaging (**Fig. 12**). The lesions fill by IV contrast from outside in and their size varies with the amount of energy deposited.[63] Thus DE-MR imaging has strong potential to follow-up on the distribution and progression of the ablation lesions.[64,65] It can, for example, be used to identify incomplete lines of ablation and target the gaps in the ablation lines during redo procedures.[66]

DE-MR imaging can also be used to assess local fibrosis in the left atrium before ablation, a result of remodeling due to chronic atrial fibrillation.[67–69] Chronic fibrosis due to remodeling is much more subtle than fibrosis due to ablation procedures, so much lower thresholds are used to identify the fibrosis of atrial remodeling. A recent study[53] indicates that a mean of 18% of the left

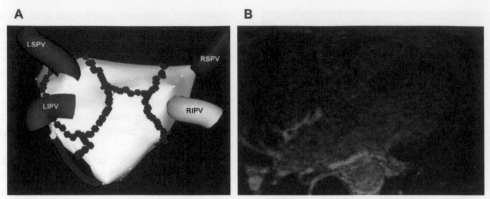

Fig. 12. Left atrial ablation therapy. (*A*) Linear ablation lesions electrically isolate the PVs. (*B*) Four-chamber long axis DE-MR image of the heart shows bright signal in the left atrium due to the ablation lines. LIPV, left inferior pulmonary vein; LSPV, left superior pulmonary vein; RIPV, right inferior pulmonary vein; RSPV, right superior pulmonary vein.

atrial wall in subjects with chronic atrial fibrillation represents fibrosis due to remodeling, and the total amount of fibrosis can be classified into 4 categories: Utah 1 (<5% fibrosis), Utah 2 (5%–20%), Utah 3 (20%–35%) and Utah 4 (>35%). These categories of fibrosis can predict the rate of recurrence after PVs and left atrial ablation therapy, with respective recurrence rates of 0%, 28%, 35%, and 56%.[53]

Intracardiac Devices

Many subjects who present with arrhythmia and who fail drug therapy receive an ICD even before they can get MR imaging to assess for the presence and distribution of myocardial scar. Implanted cardiac devices, such as pacemakers and defibrillators, used to be an absolute contraindication to MR imaging. When a subject undergoes MR imaging, there are many interactions between the MR scanner and the intracardiac devices: heating, force and torque, alteration of programming, damage to the circuitry, interference with sensing, issues with pacing (ventricular fibrillation and rapid atrial pacing), inhibition of pacing output, and threshold alteration. These interactions can lead to device failure, leading to potentially fatal arrhythmia.[70]

Leading institutions are now performing MR imaging on subjects with devices, using strict well-controlled protocols. These protocols require close cooperation between radiology and electrophysiology. At the author's institution, the protocol is as follows: (1) an electrophysiologist comes to the preparation room to interrogate the device before the MR examination, to perform some baseline measurements; (2) the device's functions to detect tachycardia and provide therapies are turned off; (3) the pacemaker is typically set to VVI mode at 40 beats per minute; (4) gentle MR

imaging is performed at 1.5 Tesla, involving gradient-echo imaging and DE imaging as well as real-time imaging if ECG gating proves difficult; (5) during the imaging, the heart rate as displayed on the pulse oxymeter is closely watched for sudden changes; (6) after the imaging session, the electrophysiologist comes to the recovery room to turn back on all the arrhythmia detection and therapy functions of the device; and (7) the device is thoroughly interrogated to assess any discrepancy from the baseline measurements.

At the author's institution, more than 400 MR examinations have been performed on subjects with devices. There was an equal split between pacemakers and implanted defibrillators. More than 60 of these examinations were cardiac MR images. Complications were minimal and included an older generation of pacemaker that went into "elective replacement interval mode" after the MR imaging but went back to normal mode after rebooting; two subjects had implanted defibrillators, and had sustained ventricular tachycardia in the magnet, that were well tolerated without ill effects.

The presence of an intracardiac device causes artifacts on the cardiac MR images. The intracardiac leads cause focal linear artifacts, which do not affect imaging of the surrounding myocardium (**Fig. 13**A). The main imaging artifact relates to the implanted control box (see **Fig. 13**B) and can mask large portions of the LV. This artifact is worse with a short distance of the control box to the LV and worse on steady-state free precession (SSFP) cine pulse sequences. The artifact also affects proper uniform nulling of the normal myocardium used for DE-MR imaging.

To optimally image myocardial scar by DE-MR imaging in subjects with intracardiac devices,

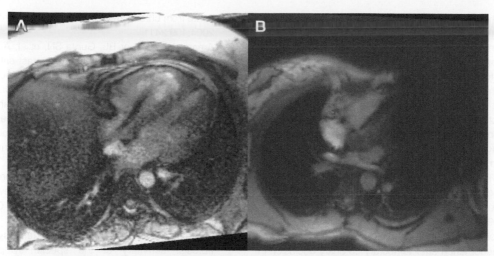

Fig. 13. Four-chamber long axis MR images in patients with intra-cardiac devices. (*A*) There is a linear area of low signal in the right atrium and right ventricle due to the artifact caused by the intracardiac metallic lead. (*B*) Large dark artifact due to the control box of the device, implanted on the left side of the chest wall. The artifact masks most of the LV.

a few options are available: (1) the bandwidth can be increased to minimize the control box artifact, which decreases echo time but also decreases the signal-to-noise ratio; (2) the control box and its overlying skin can be pulled away from the heart; (3) the anterior coils can be deactivated; (4) multiple inversion times can be sampled or a phase-sensitive inversion recovery sequence can be used; and if nothing else works, (5) postcontrast cine sequences can be used to evaluate DE.

SUMMARY

MR imaging can assess multiple facets of the heart, including anatomy, function, perfusion, flow, coronary anatomy, and scar. In the context of cardiac electrophysiology, MR imaging can be especially useful. Although anatomic and functional imaging has been routinely used for risk stratification purposes, many subjects with preserved LV function present potentially fatal arrhythmia, whereas most subjects with depressed LV function do not present significant arrhythmia. DE-MR imaging can identify the size, transmurality, and pattern of distribution of scar, which can act as arrhythmogenic substrate, as well as microvascular obstruction and associated edema. Both the size of the scar and the size of the scar border zone correlate with the risk of arrhythmia and SCD. MR imaging can thus eventually provide a much more precise risk stratification strategy compared with surrogate markers, such as LV function, because it is based on direct visualization of the arrhythmogenic substrate. MR imaging can also prove useful for high-resolution mapping of the scar, and complement EAM, especially for the identification of

intramural scar or in subjects with difficult access to the myocardium via catheter. MR imaging can also prove useful to assess left atrial scar due to chronic remodeling and to predict and follow-up the result of cardiac ablation therapy and to direct therapy during repeated procedures. Finally, many subjects with arrhythmia receive an ICD before proper imaging of myocardial scar can be performed. Strict protocols now enables imaging of these patients by MRI after implantation of an intracardiac device.

REFERENCES

1. Goldenberg I, Vyas AK, Hall WJ, et al. Risk stratification for primary implantation of a cardioverter-defibrillator in patients with ischemic left ventricular dysfunction. J Am Coll Cardiol 2008;51:288.
2. de Vreede-Swagemakers JJ, Gorgels AP, Dubois-Arbouw WI, et al. Out-of-hospital cardiac arrest in the 1990's: a population-based study in the Maastricht area on incidence, characteristics and survival. J Am Coll Cardiol 1997;30:1500.
3. Moss AJ, Zareba W, Hall WJ, et al. Prophylactic implantation of a defibrillator in patients with myocardial infarction and reduced ejection fraction. N Engl J Med 2002;346:877.
4. Bardy GH, Lee KL, Mark DB, et al. Amiodarone or an implantable cardioverter defibrillator for congestive heart failure. N Engl J Med 2005;352:225.
5. Zipes DP, Wellens HJ. Sudden cardiac death. Circulation 1998;98:2334.
6. Strauss DG, Wu KC. Imaging myocardial scar and arrhythmic risk prediction—a role for the electrocardiogram? J Electrocardiol 2009;42:138, e1–138, e8.

7. Arheden H, Saeed M, Higgins CB, et al. Measurement of the distribution volume of gadopentetate dimeglumine at echo-planar MR imaging to quantify myocardial infarction: comparison with 99mTc-DTPA autoradiography in rats. Radiology 1999;211:698.

8. Arheden H, Saeed M, Higgins CB, et al. Reperfused rat myocardium subjected to various durations of ischemia: estimation of the distribution volume of contrast material with echo-planar MR imaging. Radiology 2000;215:520.

9. Kim RJ, Chen EL, Lima JA, et al. Myocardial Gd-DTPA kinetics determine MRI contrast enhancement and reflect the extent and severity of myocardial injury after acute reperfused infarction. Circulation 1996;94:3318.

10. Kloner RA, Ganote CE, Jennings RB. The "no-reflow" phenomenon after temporary coronary occlusion in the dog. J Clin Invest 1974;54:1496.

11. Fieno DS, Hillenbrand HB, Rehwald WG, et al. Infarct resorption, compensatory hypertrophy, and differing patterns of ventricular remodeling following myocardial infarctions of varying size. J Am Coll Cardiol 2004;43:2124.

12. Fishbein MC, Maclean D, Maroko PR. The histopathologic evolution of myocardial infarction. Chest 1978;73:843.

13. Pennell DJ, Sechtem UP, Higgins CB, et al. Clinical indications for cardiovascular magnetic resonance (CMR): consensus panel report. Eur Heart J 2004;25:1940.

14. Carlsson M, Arheden H, Higgins CB, et al. Magnetic resonance imaging as a potential gold standard for infarct quantification. J Electrocardiol 2008;41:614–20.

15. Wagner A, Mahrholdt H, Thomson L, et al. Effects of time, dose, and inversion time for acute myocardial infarct size measurements based on magnetic resonance imaging-delayed contrast enhancement. J Am Coll Cardiol 2006;47:2027.

16. Simonetti O, Kim R, Fieno D, et al. An improved MR imaging technique for the visualization of myocardial infarction. Radiology 2001;218:215.

17. Kellman P, Arai AE, McVeigh ER, et al. Phase-sensitive inversion recovery for detecting myocardial infarction using gadolinium-delayed hyperenhancement. Magn Reson Med 2002;47:372–83.

18. Weber OM, Martin AJ, Higgins CB. Whole-heart steady-state free precession coronary artery magnetic resonance angiography. Magn Reson Med 2003;50(6):1223–8.

19. Bogaert J, Kalantzi M, Rademakers FE, et al. Determinants and impact of microvascular obstruction in successfully reperfused ST-segment elevation myocardial infarction. Assessment by magnetic resonance imaging. Eur Radiol 2007;17:2572.

20. Abdel-Aty H, Zagrosek A, Schulz-Menger J, et al. Delayed enhancement and T2-weighted cardiovascular magnetic resonance imaging differentiate acute from chronic myocardial infarction. Circulation 2004;109:2411.

21. Amado LC, Gerber BL, Gupta SN, et al. Accurate and objective infarct sizing by contrast-enhanced magnetic resonance imaging in a canine myocardial infarction model. J Am Coll Cardiol 2004;44:2383.

22. Hsu LY, Natanzon A, Kellman P, et al. Quantitative myocardial infarction on delayed enhancement MRI. Part I: animal validation of an automated feature analysis and combined thresholding infarct sizing algorithm. J Magn Reson Imaging 2006;23:298.

23. Kim RJ, Fieno DS, Parrish TB, et al. Relationship of MRI delayed contrast enhancement to irreversible injury, infarct age, and contractile function. Circulation 1999;100:1992.

24. Bongartz G, Kucharczyk W. Nephrogenic systemic fibrosis: summary of the special symposium. J Magn Reson Imaging 2007;26:1179–81.

25. Witschey WR, Pilla JJ, Ferrari G, et al. Rotating frame spin lattice relaxation in a swine model of chronic, left ventricular myocardial infarction. Magn Reson Med 2010;64:1453–60.

26. Stevenson WG, Delacretaz E. Radiofrequency catheter ablation of ventricular tachycardia. Heart 2000; 84:553–9.

27. Desjardins B, Crawford T, Good E, et al. Infarct architecture and characteristics on delayed enhanced magnetic resonance imaging and electroanatomic mapping in patients with postinfarction ventricular arrhythmia. Heart Rhythm 2009;6:644–51.

28. Desjardins B, Morady F, Bogun F. Effect of epicardial fat on electroanatomical mapping and epicardial catheter ablation. J Am Coll Cardiol 2010;56:1320–7.

29. Yan AT, Shayne AJ, Brown KA, et al. Characterization of the peri-infarct zone by contrast-enhanced cardiac magnetic resonance imaging is a powerful predictor of post-myocardial infarction mortality. Circulation 2006;114:32.

30. Schmidt A, Azevedo CF, Cheng A, et al. Infarct tissue heterogeneity by magnetic resonance imaging identifies enhanced cardiac arrhythmia susceptibility in patients with left ventricular dysfunction. Circulation 2007;115:2006.

31. Bogun F, Desjardins B, Crawford T, et al. Post-infarction ventricular arrhythmias originating in papillary muscles. J Am Coll Cardiol 2008;51:1794–802.

32. Nazarian S, Bluemke DA, Lardo AC, et al. Magnetic resonance assessment of the substrate for inducible ventricular tachycardia in nonischemic cardiomyopathy. Circulation 2005;112:2821.

33. Mahrholdt H, Wagner A, Judd RM, et al. Delayed enhancement cardiovascular magnetic resonance assessment of non-ischaemic cardiomyopathies. Eur Heart J 2005;26:1461.

34. O'Hanlon R, Prasad SK, Pennell DJ. Evaluation of nonischemic cardiomyopathies using cardiovascular magnetic resonance. J Nucl Cardiol 2008;15:400.

35. Bolick DR, Hackel DB, Reimer KA, et al. Quantitative analysis of myocardial infarct structure in patients with ventricular tachycardia. Circulation 1986;74: 1266–79.

36. Mann DL, Bristow MR. Mechanisms and models in heart failure: the biomechanical model and beyond. Circulation 2005;111:2837.

37. Macedo R, Schmidt A, Rochitte CE, et al. MRI to assess arrhythmia and cardiomyopathies. J Magn Reson Imaging 2006;24:1197.

38. Assomull RG, Prasad SK, Lyne J, et al. Cardiovascular magnetic resonance, fibrosis, and prognosis in dilated cardiomyopathy. J Am Coll Cardiol 2006; 48:1977.

39. Wu KC, Weiss RG, Thiemann DR, et al. Late gadolinium enhancement by cardiovascular magnetic resonance heralds an adverse prognosis in nonischemic cardiomyopathy. J Am Coll Cardiol 2008; 51:2414.

40. Maron BJ, Spirito P. Implantable defibrillators and prevention of sudden death in hypertrophic cardiomyopathy. J Cardiovasc Electrophysiol 2008;19:1118.

41. Shirani J, Pick R, Roberts WC, et al. Morphology and significance of the left ventricular collagen network in young patients with hypertrophic cardiomyopathy and sudden cardiac death. J Am Coll Cardiol 2000; 35:36.

42. Moon JC, McKenna WJ, McCrohon JA, et al. Toward clinical risk assessment in hypertrophic cardiomyopathy with gadolinium cardiovascular magnetic resonance. J Am Coll Cardiol 2003;41:1561.

43. Adabag AS, Maron BJ, Appelbaum E, et al. Occurrence and frequency of arrhythmias in hypertrophic cardiomyopathy in relation to delayed enhancement on cardiovascular magnetic resonance. J Am Coll Cardiol 2008;51:1369.

44. Moon JC, Sachdev B, Elkington AG, et al. Gadolinium enhanced cardiovascular magnetic resonance in Anderson-Fabry disease. Evidence for a disease specific abnormality of the myocardial interstitium. Eur Heart J 2003;24:2151.

45. Mahrholdt H, Goedecke C, Wagner A, et al. Cardiovascular magnetic resonance assessment of human myocarditis: a comparison to histology and molecular pathology. Circulation 2004;109:1250.

46. Friedrich MG, Strohm O, Schulz-Menger J, et al. Contrast media-enhanced magnetic resonance imaging visualizes myocardial changes in the course of viral myocarditis. Circulation 1998;97:1802.

47. Shammas RL, Movahed A. Sarcoidosis of the heart. Clin Cardiol 1993;16:462.

48. Silverman KJ, Hutchins GM, Bulkley BH. Cardiac sarcoid: a clinicopathologic study of 84 unselected patients with systemic sarcoidosis. Circulation 1978;58:1204.

49. Schulz-Menger J, Wassmuth R, Abdel-Aty H, et al. Patterns of myocardial inflammation and scarring in sarcoidosis as assessed by cardiovascular magnetic resonance. Heart 2006;92:399.

50. Smedema JP, Snoep G, van Kroonenburgh MP, et al. Evaluation of the accuracy of gadolinium-enhanced cardiovascular magnetic resonance in the diagnosis of cardiac sarcoidosis. J Am Coll Cardiol 2005;45: 1683.

51. Rochitte CE, Oliveira PF, Andrade JM, et al. Myocardial delayed enhancement by magnetic resonance imaging in patients with Chagas' disease: a marker of disease severity. J Am Coll Cardiol 2005;46:1553.

52. Hart RG, Palacio S, Pearce LA. Atrial fibrillation, stroke, and acute antithrombotic therapy: analysis of randomized clinical trials. Stroke 2002;33:2722–7.

53. Akoum N, Daccarett M, Mcgann C, et al. Atrial fibrosis helps select the appropriate patient and strategy in catheter ablation of atrial fibrillation: a DE-MRI guided approach. J Cardiovasc Electrophysiol 2011;22:16–22.

54. Cronin P, Kelly AM, Desjardins B, et al. Normative analysis of pulmonary vein drainage patterns on multidetector CT with measurements of pulmonary vein ostial diameter and distance to first bifurcation. Acad Radiol 2007;14:178–88.

55. Hof I, Chilukuri K, Arbab-Zadeh A, et al. Does left atrial volume and pulmonary venous anatomy predict the outcome of catheter ablation of atrial fibrillation? J Cardiovasc Electrophysiol 2009;20: 1005–10.

56. Kurotobi T, Iwakura K, Inoue K, et al. The significance of the shape of the left atrial roof as a novel index for determining the electrophysiological and structural characteristics in patients with atrial fibrillation. Europace 2011;13:803–8.

57. Lemola K, Sneider M, Desjardins B, et al. Computed tomographic analysis of the anatomy of the left atrium and the esophagus: implications for left atrial catheter ablation. Circulation 2004;110:3655–60.

58. Li YG, Yang M, Li Y, et al. Spatial relationship between left atrial roof or superior pulmonary veins and bronchi or pulmonary arteries by dual-source computed tomography: implication for preventing injury of bronchi and pulmonary arteries during atrial fibrillation ablation. Europace 2011;13(6): 809–14.

59. Horton R, Di Biase L, Reddy V, et al. Locating the right phrenic nerve by imaging the right pericardiophrenic artery with computerized tomographic angiography: implications for balloon-based procedures. Heart Rhythm 2010;7:937–41.

60. Dong J, Calkins H, Solomon SB, et al. Integrated electroanatomic mapping with three-dimensional computed tomographic images for real-time guided ablations. Circulation 2006;113:186–94.

61. De Ponti R, Marazzi R, Lumia D, et al. Role of three-dimensional imaging integration in atrial fibrillation ablation. World J Cardiol 2010;2:215–22.

62. Okada T, Yamada T, Murakami Y, et al. Prevalence and severity of left atrial edema detected by electron beam tomography early after pulmonary vein ablation. J Am Coll Cardiol 2007;49:1436–42.

63. Dickfeld T, Kato R, Zviman M, et al. Characterization of radiofrequency ablation lesions with gadolinium-enhanced cardiovascular magnetic resonance imaging. J Am Coll Cardiol 2006;47:370–8.

64. Peters DC, Wylie JV, Hauser TH, et al. Detection of pulmonary vein and left atrial scar after catheter ablation with three-dimensional navigator-gated delayed enhancement MR imaging: initial experience. Radiology 2007;243:690–5.

65. Oakes RS, Badger TJ, Kholmovski EG, et al. Detection and quantification of left atrial structural remodeling with delayed-enhancement magnetic resonance imaging in patients with atrial fibrillation. Circulation 2009;119:1758–67.

66. McGann CJ, Kholmovski EG, Oakes RS, et al. New magnetic resonance imaging-based method for defining the extent of left atrial wall injury after the ablation of atrial fibrillation. J Am Coll Cardiol 2008; 52:1263–71.

67. Ausma J, Wijffels M, Thone F, et al. Structural changes of atrial myocardium due to sustained atrial fibrillation in the goat. Circulation 1997;96:3157–63.

68. Allessie M, Ausma J, Schotten U. Electrical, contractile and structural remodeling during atrial fibrillation. Cardiovasc Res 2002;54:230–6.

69. Casaclang-Verzosa G, Gersh BJ, Tsang TS. Structural and functional remodeling of the left atrium: clinical and therapeutic implications for atrial fibrillation. J Am Coll Cardiol 2008;51:1–11.

70. Levine GN, Gomes AS, Arai AE, et al. Safety of magnetic resonance imaging in patients with cardiovascular devices. Circulation 2007;116:2878–91.

Index

Note: Page numbers of article titles are in **boldface** type.

A

Amyloidosis, MR imaging for, 481
Arrhythmogenic right ventricular dysplasia, MR imaging for, 483–484
Atherosclerosis
  PET for
    for calcium scoring, 444–445
    with inflammation, **417–420**
  PET/CT for, 410–414, **421–429**
    evaluation of response to therapy, 424–425
    prognostic use of, 426–427
    quantification of, 421–426
Atrial fibrillation, radiofrequency ablation for
  CT angiography in, 447
  MR imaging in, 496–498
Autoimmune diseases, MR imaging for, 484–485

B

Biopsy, for sarcoidosis, 404

C

Calcification. *See* Atherosclerosis.
Calcium scoring, CT angiography for, 444–445
Cardiac CT angiography, **441–452**
Cardiac MR imaging. *See* MR imaging.
Cardiac PET. *See* PET.
Cardiac resynchronization therapy, 464
Cardiomyopathy, MR imaging for, 493–496
  nonischemic, **475–487**
    decision making for, 476–478
    examples of, 478–486
    late gadinolinium enhancement in, 475–477
    myocardial edema in, 476
Chagas disease, MR imaging for, 485
Coronary artery(ies)
  anatomy of, CT angiography for, 447–449
  anomalies of, CT angiography for, 449
  atherosclerosis of. *See* Atherosclerosis.
  evaluation of. *See* CT angiography.
Coronary artery bypass graft evaluation, CT angiography for, 445
Coronary Artery Surgery Study registry, 387
CT
  during ventricular tachycardia ablation, 398–399
  for ischemic heart disease, 459
  PET with, for atherosclerosis, **409–415, 421–429**

CT angiography, **441–452**
  conventional, 443–444
  evolution of, 441–442
  for calcium scoring, 443–444
  for cardiac conditions, **441–452**
  for coronary artery anatomy, 447–449
  for coronary artery anomalies, 449
  for coronary artery bypass graft evaluation, 444–447
  for coronary artery evaluation, 442–443
  for left ventricular function, 444
  for myocardial perfusion, 434–435
  for myocardial viability, 447
  for stent evaluation, 445–446
  for venous mapping, 447
  indications for, 449
  protocol for, 442

D

Dilated cardiomyopathy, MR imaging for, 484
Dobutamine stress test, with MR imaging, 461–462
Drug-induced cardiomyopathy, MR imaging for, 484

E

Echocardiography
  for myocardial viability, 386
  for sarcoidosis, 404
Electroanatomic mapping, for myocardial scar, 492–493
Electrocardiography, for sarcoidosis, 404
Electrophysiology, in myocardial scar, MR imaging with, 490–493
Endomyocardial biopsy, for sarcoidosis, 404
Eosinophilic heart disease, MR imaging for, 481–482
Exercise stress test, with MR imaging, 462

F

FDG
  PET
    during ventricular tachycardia ablation, **393–402**
    for atherosclerosis, **409–415, 417–429**
    for myocardial perfusion, **431–439**
    for myocardial viability, **383–391**
    for sarcoidosis, **403–408**
  SPECT, for myocardial viability, 386

PET Clin 6 (2011) 503–505
doi:10.1016/S1556-8598(11)00123-4

Printed and bound by CPI Group (UK) Ltd, Croydon, CR0 4YY
03/10/2024
01040358-0013